# Your Heart Belongs to You

Body Dynamics Volume Two

Marsena Shane

BLACK BED SHEET

**Your Heart Belongs to You**
**(Body Dynamics Volume Two)**
A Black Bed Sheet/Diverse Media Book
Revised and updated
Second Edition, April 2026



This is a work of nonfiction. The information provided is for educational purposes and should not replace professional medical advice. Always consult a physician before beginning any new exercise or diet program.

# Your Heart Belongs to You

**A Black Bed Sheet/Diverse Media Book**
**Sacramento, CA**

## Also by Marsena Shane:

The East Way to Great Legs
(Body Dynamics Volume 1)

Sweet Dreams, Lady Moon

June Park

Nancy: A Reagan Biography

The Martian Coal Miner

The Jupiter Possums

To my readers, thank you for embarking on this journey toward better health with me. Your commitment to self-improvement is my greatest inspiration. To my editor, your sharp eye and dedication to preserving the unique 1990s spirit of this book were invaluable. I also want to thank my beta readers, whose early feedback ensured that these routines and insights would resonate with everyone.

To my family and friends, thank you for your endless patience and for cheering me on during the long hours of research and writing. Your belief in this project never wavered. Finally, to the healthcare professionals who continue to advance our understanding of the human heart—thank you for your tireless work. This book is a tribute to the power of the human spirit and the strength of the heart that sustains us all.

Note: This book is revised and updated from its original Critic's Choice Paperbacks 1990 publication. The 1990s were an important time for for medical enlightenment with a far greater awareness of physical fitness than ever before, so the revision maintains and celebrates its 1990s origins.

# Chapter 1
# The Pulse of History: Ancient Hearts to Modern Beats

You are holding the key to your future right now. It is right there, beating inside your chest, steady and relentless. You might not think about it often, or maybe you only think about it when you are winded from a flight of stairs, but that heart of yours is the most important piece of equipment you will ever own. It is more than just a pump. It is the very center of your existence, the engine that drives every dream, every walk in the park, and every long day at the office. Today, we are starting a journey to reclaim that engine. We are going to take it out of the garage, tune it up, and make sure it runs for a very long time. You see, your heart belongs to you, and it is about time you started acting like the owner of such a high-performance machine. This is not just about avoiding problems; it is about reaching a level of vitality you might have forgotten was even possible.

### The Heart of the Matter

When you stop to consider the sheer power of the human heart, it is enough to make you sit up a little straighter. This muscular organ, roughly the size of your two fists clenched on strike. It works while you sleep, while you eat, and while you watch your favorite sitcoms. It pushes gallons of blood through miles of vessels, ensuring that every single cell in your body gets the oxygen and nutrients it needs to thrive. But for too many of us, the heart is a mystery. We treat it like a black box—something that just works until it doesn't. That ends today. We are going to demystify this incredible organ and give you the tools to manage it with confidence and authority.

Understanding your heart is the first step toward a longer, more energetic life. We are living in an era where we have more information than ever before about how to stay fit, yet we often feel more disconnected from our bodies than our ancestors did. They saw the heart as the seat of the soul, the place where courage and love resided. While we now have the medical technology to see it as a biological machine, we should not lose that sense of wonder. Your heart is both a mechanical marvel and the emotional core of your being. By the time you finish this book, you will by looking at the actual hardware that makes your life possible.

### Anatomy 101: The Engine, A House with Four Rooms

These rooms are called chambers, and they work in a perfectly timed sequence to keep everything moving. The top ventricle. These are the powerful pumping rooms that send the blood back out into the world of your body. It is a simple setup, but the coordination required to keep it running is nothing short of miraculous.

The right side of your heart is the staging area for blood that has already been through your body. This blood is low on oxygen and needs a refill. It enters the right atrium, drops down into the right ventricle, and then gets pushed out to the lungs. In the lungs, the blood picks up fresh oxygen and gets rid of carbon dioxide. Once it is refreshed and bright red again, it travels back to the left side of the heart. The left atrium receives this oxygen-rich blood and passes it to the left ventricle. Now, the left ventricle is the real powerhouse of the group. It has thick, muscular walls because it has to generate enough pressure to blast that blood all the way down to your toes and all the way up to your brain. This constant cycle—receive, pump to lungs, receive, pump to body—is the rhythm of your life.

Between these chambers are valves. Think of them as one-way doors. They make sure that the blood only flows in one direction. "Lub" is the sound of the valves between the atria and ventricles closing, and the "dub" is the sound of the valves leading out of the heart closing. If those doors are working right, your circulation is efficient. If they get those "doors" and "pipes" clear so the engine does not have to strain. When your heart is healthy, the blood flows like a clear mountain stream. When it is not, it is more like trying to push sludge through a straw. We are going to stick with the mountain stream, thank you very much.

### The 90s Wellness Strategy: Your Baseline Vitality Profile

Before we can improve your health, we need to know exactly where you are gas gauge is your resting heart rate. This is the number of times your heart beats per minute when you are completely relaxed. It is one of the most powerful indicators of your overall cardiovascular fitness. Generally speaking, a lower resting heart rate means a more efficient heart. Athletes often have very low resting heart rates because their hearts are so strong that they can move a large volume of blood with very little effort. For the rest of us, getting that number down is a primary goal of our fitness journey.

We are going to establish what I call your **Baseline Vitality Profile**. This is your personal data set that will prove to you that your hard work is paying off. To do this, you need to learn how to take your pulse manually. Forget the fancy gadgets for a moment; there is something deeply empowering about feeling your own life force with your own fingers. The best place to find it is the radial pulse, located on your wrist. Here is how you do it:

1. Turn one hand palm up.
2. Use the index and middle fingers of your other hand (never use your thumb, as it has a pulse of its own that can confuse your count).
3. Place those two fingers on the thumb side of your wrist, just below the base of the hand.
4. Press lightly until you feel the rhythmic thumping. It might take a second to find the right spot, so be patient.
5. Once you have a steady beat, look at a watch with a second hand. Count the beats for a full sixty seconds.

That number is your resting heart rate. For the best results, you should take this measurement first thing in the morning, before you even get out of bed. Caffeine, stress, and even a brisk walk to the kitchen can raise the number and give you an inaccurate baseline. I want you to start a daily log in a dedicated notebook. Write down the date and your resting heart rate every single morning. Over the next few weeks and months, as we implement the diet and exercise strategies in this book, you are going to see that number start to drop. That is the feeling of success. That is your heart getting stronger and more efficient. It is your first real piece of evidence that you are taking control of, the most important part of the human being. They believed it was the seat of intelligence, emotion, and memory. When they mummified their dead, they threw away the brain—literally hooked it out through the nose and discarded it—because they thought it was just a cooling organ of no real use. But the heart? They left the heart inside the body. They believed that in the afterlife, the heart would be weighed against the feather of Ma'at, the goddess of truth. If your heart was heavy with sin, you were in trouble. This shows us that the connection between the heart and our "true self" is thousands of years old.

As we move into the era of the Ancient Greeks, the understanding shifted but remained somewhat mystical. Great thinkers like Galen believed the body was governed by four "humors" or fluids: blood, phlegm, yellow bile, and black bile. They thought the heart was a furnace that produced heat for the body and that the blood the accepted "truth." People believed that blood was constantly being created and then consumed by the body, like fuel in a fire. It is a bit wild to think about now, but this shows how hard it is to see the truth when you don't have the right tools or the right mindset.

The real breakthrough came in the seventeenth century with a man named William Harvey. Harvey an hour and realized that there was no way the body could produce that much blood from food every day. The math just didn't add up. He concluded that the blood must be moving in a circle—circulating. This was a it as a system that could be studied, understood, and eventually, improved. Today, we stand on the shoulders of these thinkers. We know the heart is a pump, but we can still respect the Egyptian idea that it is the center of our lives. When you take care of your heart, you are taking care of your "self" in every sense of the word.

## Why Knowledge is Your Best Defense

You might be wondering why we are spending time on history and anatomy. Why not just jump straight into the push-ups and the salads? Well, let me tell you, knowledge is the foundation of motivation. If I just tell you to run, you might do it for a week. But if you understand that running is strengthening the muscular walls of your left ventricle, making it more efficient at delivering oxygen to your brain so you can lot easier.

We are also fighting against a lot of modern misconceptions. Many people think that heart health is something you only need to worry about when you get gray hair. That is a dangerous mistake. The habits that lead to a healthy heart—or a diseased one—start right now, regardless of your age. The plaque that clogs arteries doesn't show up overnight; it is the result of years of choices. By taking charge of your heart health today, you are performing a revolutionary act of self-care. You are deciding that you are not going to be a statistic. You are deciding that you want to be there for your grandkids' graduations, that you want to be active in your golden years, and that you want to feel great every single morning between now and then.

This journey is about more than just numbers on a scale or a pulse count. It is about a feeling of vitality. Vitality is that spark of energy that makes you want to get out of bed and tackle the day. It is the ability to play a game of catch without getting winded. It is the confidence that comes from knowing your body is strong. Throughout this book, I am going to be your coach, your teacher, and your biggest cheerleader. We are going to do this together, one step at a time, one beat at a time. The road to a better heart is paved with small, consistent actions. It is not about a radical overhaul that you quit after three days; it is about building a lifestyle that you love.

**Your Action Plan: Day One**

It is time to put some skin in the game. I don't want you to just read this and put the book down. I want you to take action right now. We are going to start small, but these five steps are the foundation of everything that follows. Grab a pen and let's make a commitment to your future self.

1. **Buy a dedicated notebook.** This is your Heart Log. It doesn't have to be fancy—a simple spiral notebook will do. This is where you will record your morning resting heart rate, your exercise minutes, and your thoughts on your progress. Treating this like a formal project makes it real.

2. **Practice finding your pulse.** I want you to be able to find your radial pulse within five seconds. Practice on yourself, practice on your spouse, practice on your kids. Get comfortable with the feeling of that rhythm. It is the sound of your life, and you should be familiar with it.

3. **List three personal reasons for this journey.** Why are you doing this? Maybe you want to lose twenty pounds. Maybe you want to stop feeling so tired in the afternoon. Maybe you saw a family member struggle with heart issues and you want a different path. Write these three things on the first page of your Heart Log. When things get tough, these reasons will be your fuel.

4. **Remove one high-sodium snack from your pantry.** We aren't overhauling your entire kitchen today, but we are

making a statement. Salt makes your body hold onto water and raises your blood pressure, making your heart work harder. Pick one bag of salty chips or a can of processed soup and get it out of the house. It is a symbolic first strike in the war for your health.

5. **Walk for ten minutes.** Right now, or as soon as you finish this chapter, go outside and walk for ten minutes. This isn't a marathon. It's a celebration. You are telling your heart: "Hey, we're back in business." Pay attention to how the air feels in your lungs and how your legs feel as they move. You are alive, and that is a wonderful thing.

You have taken the first step on a path that leads to a stronger, more vibrant version of yourself. The heart is a resilient organ. It wants to be healthy. It wants to work for you. All it needs is a little bit of cooperation and the right kind of fuel. In the chapters ahead, we will dive deeper into the myths of heart health, the best ways to eat for a strong ticker, and exercise routines that are actually fun. But for today, be proud of yourself. You've acknowledged that your heart belongs to you, and you've started the process of taking it back. Keep that notebook handy, and I will see you in the next chapter where we'll start busting some of the biggest myths that might be holding you back. Your heart is ready. Are you?

Remember, this is not a race; it is a steady climb. You might have ignored your heart for the last decade, but that doesn't mean the next decade has to be the same. Every morning you wake up is a new opportunity to give your heart what it needs. Whether you are twenty-five or sixty-five, the benefits of heart-smart living are available to you starting right this second. We are going to look at the food you eat, the way you move, and even the way you think, because all of it affects that pump in your chest. You are the captain of this ship, and your heart is the engine. Let's make sure it's the most powerful engine on the water. Stay motivated, stay curious, and most importantly, stay active. Your journey has officially begun.

# Chapter 2
# Myths, Legends, and the Pump of Life

Say, you want to live longer? How about taking steps to improve your body through diet and exercise and an understanding of your heart as well as the human heart altogether throughout the ages? Well you've come to the right place, let me tell you. In our last session, we looked at the basics of the four chambers and why you need to start a heart log. Now, we are going to dive into the stories we tell ourselves about our health. You see, there is a lot of misinformation floating around out there in the world, and some of it is as old as the hills. If you are going to be the master of your own cardiovascular destiny, you have to be able to separate the cold, hard facts from the tall tales. We are going to look at the myths that hold us back and the actual biological structures that keep us moving forward.

## The Heart of the Matter

Do not let old wives' tales keep you from the truth about your health. We have all heard them at some point or another. Maybe your grandfather told you that a glass of salty broth is the only way to cure a dizzy spell, or perhaps you grew up believing that if you can't feel your heart hammering against your ribs like a trapped bird, you aren't actually getting a good workout. These ideas might seem harmless, but they create a mental fog that makes it hard to see what your body actually needs. When we believe things that aren't true, we make choices that can actually hinder our progress. It is time to clear the air and look at the heart for what it really is: a high-performance machine that requires precision care, not guesswork and folklore.

The truth is that many people are actually afraid of their hearts. They think of the heart as a fragile thing, something that might "snap" if they push it too hard or "break" if they experience too much stress. While the heart is certainly affected by our emotions and our physical efforts, it is also incredibly resilient. It is built to work, and it is built to last. By dismantling the myths that suggest otherwise, we empower ourselves to push further and today. This isn't just about learning new information; it's about unlearning the bad information that has been slowing you down for years. Let's get the facts straight so we can get your heart in the best shape of its life.

### Anatomy 101: The Protective Shield

When we talk about the heart, we usually focus on the muscles and the valves—the parts that do the heavy lifting of pumping blood. But there is another part of the system that is just as important, even if it doesn't get as much press. I am talking about the **pericardium**. This is the protective sac that surrounds your heart, and it plays a vital role in keeping your internal engine safe and running smoothly. Think of it like the casing on a high-end car engine. It isn't the part that makes the car go, but without it, the engine would be exposed to the elements and would likely overheat or seize up in no time at all.

The pericardium is a double-layered membrane. The outer layer is tough and fibrous, which helps to keep the heart in place within the chest cavity. It prevents the heart from moving around too much when you are jumping, running, or just living your life. It also acts as a physical barrier against infections that might be floating around in the rest of your body. The inner layer is much smoother and more delicate. Between these two layers is a very small amount of fluid—pericardial fluid—which acts as a lubricant. Every time your heart beats, it expands and contracts. This fluid ensures that there is no friction between the heart and the surrounding structures. Without this lubrication, every single heartbeat would be a painful, grinding experience. Your heart literally floats in a tiny sea of protection.

Understanding the pericardium helps us realize that heart health is about more than just the strength of the pump. It is also about the health can cause sharp chest pain and make it difficult for the heart to fill with blood. This is why we focus on total body wellness. When you eat a diet high in antioxidants and stay hydrated, you are nourishing that protective sac and the fluid inside it. You are making sure that your heart has a comfortable, frictionless place to do its job. It is a reminder that every part of your anatomy has a purpose, and when we take care of the "shell," we are also taking care of the "engine."

### The 90s Wellness Strategy: The Myth-Buster Routine

Now, let's get down to the business of busting some myths with a real-world strategy you can use every time you lace up your sneakers. One of the most dangerous ideas in the fitness world is the phrase: **"no pain, no gain."** You've heard it at the gym, you've seen it on television, and you might even have it tattooed on your brain. But let me tell you something: your heart does not want you to be in pain. Sharp, stabbing pain is your body's way of screaming that something is wrong. When people believe they have to suffer to get healthy, they often overdo it, leading to injuries or burnout that stops their progress cold. The centerpiece of our 90s Wellness Strategy this week is the **Talk Test**. This is a simple, foolproof way to measure your exercise intensity without needing a fancy computer strapped to your chest. The idea is that if you are working in full sentences without gasping for air, you are in the "sweet spot." You are challenging your heart enough to make it stronger, but you aren't pushing it into the red zone where you risk overexertion. If you find is no prize for being the most breathless person in the park.

Another myth we need to tackle is the idea that "light activity" doesn't count. Some people think that if they aren't dripping with sweat and gasping for breath, they aren't actually helping their hearts. That is simply not true. Consistency is much more important than intensity. A brisk fifteen-minute walk every day is infinitely better for your cardiovascular system than a grueling hour-long run once a month. When you engage in light activity, you are training your heart to be more efficient at a baseline level. You are also keeping your blood vessels flexible and your pericardium lubricated. By using the Talk Test, you can ensure that you are staying in that productive range where you are doing the most good for your body without the unnecessary risk of "pushing through the pain."

### The Heart Through Time: Courtly Love and Medical Delays

To understand why we still struggle with myths today, it helps to look back at how we viewed the heart in the past. If we look at the Middle Ages, we see a time when the heart became much more than a biological organ; it became the ultimate symbol of **courtly love**. This was the era of knights and ladies, of poets literature, it actually caused a significant delay in our medical understanding of how the body works. When people view an organ as a mystical vessel for the soul and the seat of all romantic passion, they are much less likely to treat it as a machine that needs maintenance.

During this period, the heart was often depicted in art and poetry as the place where the "true self" resided. If a knight was brave, it was because he had a "lion's heart." If a lady was kind, she had a "heart of gold." This romanticized view was so powerful that it overshadowed the actual physical reality of the heart. Physicians of the time were often hesitant to study the heart too closely for fear of disturbing the divine or the emotional core of the person. This meant that while we were getting very good at writing sonnets about the heart, we were making almost no progress in understanding how to fix it when it stopped working correctly. We were stuck in a loop of metaphors while people were still suffering from very real, very physical ailments.

This history is important because those if the muscle actually cracks, or we say someone has a "cold heart" as if the temperature of the blood has changed. These metaphors are beautiful, but they can be distracting. When we think of the heart primarily as an emotional symbol, we might forget that it is also a muscle that needs fiber, oxygen, and regular movement. By acknowledging the Middle Ages' contribution to our romantic history, we can also recognize the need to move beyond it. We can appreciate the poetry of the heart while still focusing on the hard science of its survival. Your heart can be the seat of your love and the engine of your life at the same time, but only if you keep it healthy enough to keep beating.

## Label Reading: The Hidden Heart-Haters

As we move into the practical side of our journey, we have to talk about what you are putting into your body. In the 90s, we are seeing a massive surge in "diet" foods and "low-fat" options. You walk down the grocery store aisle and see labels everywhere screaming about being "Heart Healthy" or "Light." But here is the catch: just because something is low in fat doesn't mean it's good for your heart. This is another major myth we need to bust right now. Many manufacturers, in an effort to make their low-fat products taste good, loaded them up with something far worse: **hidden sugars**.

When you take the fat out of a cookie or a salad dressing, you often lose the flavor and the texture that makes it satisfying. To fix this, food companies often add high amounts of sugar or high-fructose corn syrup. While you might be avoiding the fat, you are spiking your blood sugar, which leads to inflammation and weight gain—both of which put, colorful claims on the front of the box. Turn that package around and look at the actual ingredients list. If sugar (or its many aliases like maltodextrin, dextrose, or sucrose) is one of the first few ingredients, put it back on the shelf.

Sodium is another hidden heart-hater that lurks in "diet" foods. To preserve these processed items and give them a kick of flavor, they are often packed with salt. As we discussed in our last chapter, salt makes your body hold onto water, which increases the volume of your blood and forces your heart to pump harder against higher pressure. It is a recipe for hypertension. When you read labels, look for the sodium content and compare it to the serving size. You might be surprised to find that your "healthy" frozen dinner has more salt than a large order of fries. By learning to read between the lines of the marketing jargon, you are taking a massive step toward protecting your heart from the hidden dangers of the modern diet.

### Your Action Plan: Taking the Reins

It is time to take everything we have discussed and turn it into action. Knowledge without application is just trivia, and we aren't here for trivia; we are here for transformation. I want you to take these three steps over the next few days to solidify your role as the commander of your own health. These aren't suggestions—they are the blueprints for your new lifestyle.

1. **Identify two health myths you grew up with.** Sit down with your Heart Log and think about the things you've always believed about your body. Do you think then write the reality next to them. For example: "Myth: No pain, no gain. Reality: The Talk Test is the best measure of a safe, effective workout." When you see these myths on paper, they lose their power over you.

2. **Perform a light 15-minute stretch to feel the pericardial flexibility.** We talked about the pericardium and how it protects your heart. I want you to spend fifteen minutes doing some very gentle upper body stretches. Reach your arms toward the sky, gently twist your torso from side to side, and take deep, full breaths that expand your ribcage. As you do; it's about connecting with the physical reality of your anatomy. Feel how your chest and lungs provide the space your heart needs to do its job.

3. **Read the labels of 'diet' foods to check for hidden sugars.** Go to your pantry right now and grab three items that are marketed as "low-fat," "diet," or "light." Read the ingredients list. Look for sugar, corn syrup, or any word ending in "-ose." Check the sodium levels too. If you find that your "healthy" snacks are actually sugar-and-salt bombs, don't beat yourself up. Just acknowledge it and make a better choice next time you are at the store. Information is your best weapon in the battle for your health.

By completing these steps, you are moving from a passive observer of your health to an active participant. You are no longer someone who just "hopes" their heart is doing okay; you are someone who knows how to check the engine, how to shield it from harm, and how to fuel it not just days. Each time you choose the Talk Test over "pushing through the pain," or fresh fruit over a "diet" snack, you are casting a vote for a longer, more vibrant life.

The human heart is an incredible piece of equipment. It has survived centuries of myths, from being the seat of the soul to being the victim of courtly love. It has endured the misconceptions of the "no pain, no gain" era and the hidden traps You have the power to change your story. You have the power to live with more energy and less fear. This is your holds. Keep your notebook close, stay active, and I will see you in the next chapter as we continue our journey toward peak vitality.

You've already made more progress than most people do in a lifetime just by showing up and being willing to learn the truth. Don't stop now. The road ahead is filled with even more discoveries that will help you fine-tune your body and sharpen your mind. Your heart is the most loyal partner you will ever have—it's time you started treating it like one. Let's keep moving, one healthy beat at a time.

# Chapter 3
## The Engine Room: Your Heart and Lungs

Imagine you just bought a brand-new, top-of-the-line sports car. The paint is shimmering, the tires are grippy, and under the hood sits a powerful engine ready to roar. You turn the key, and the engine purrs. But what happens if you clog the air intake? What if you restrict the amount of oxygen reaching that engine? It doesn't matter how much fuel you have or how strong the pistons are; without air, that car is just a very expensive piece of driveway art. Your body works the exact same way. If your heart is the engine, your lungs are the high-performance intake system. They are the two most important teammates in your body, and they are constantly passing the ball back and forth to keep you moving, thinking, and living at your peak.

When we talk about fitness in this day and age, we often focus solely on the pump—the heart. We want a lower resting heart rate and a higher stroke volume. But we have to remember that the heart is a consumer. It needs fuel to do its job, and its primary fuel is oxygen. Every time your heart beats, it is doing so using energy that was made possible by the breath you just took. If you want to maximize your cardiovascular health, you have to understand the partnership between these two organs. They are physically connected, biologically dependent, and they even share the same space in your chest cavity, protected by the same sturdy cage of ribs. They are the twin pillars of your vitality.

## The Pulmonary Loop: A Journey of Renewal

To understand how to train better, we need to take a quick look at the plumbing. Most of us think of blood as just "blood," but in reality, your circulatory system is split into two very different circuits. The first is the systemic circuit, which sends oxygen-rich blood out to your toes, your brain, and your biceps. But the second circuit—the one we are focusing on today—is the pulmonary circulation loop. This is the dedicated highway that runs exclusively between your heart and your lungs. It is a loop of constant renewal and cleaning, and it is where the real magic of life happens at a molecular level.

When your blood returns to the heart after traveling through your body, it is tired. It has dropped off its cargo of oxygen and picked up a load of carbon dioxide, which is essentially the exhaust soot of your metabolism. This blood is a dark, dull red—almost purple. It enters the right side of your heart, which acts as a staging area. From there, the heart pumps this "dirty" blood into the pulmonary arteries. Here is a fun fact for your next dinner party: the pulmonary arteries are the only arteries in the human body that carry deoxygenated blood. Usually, arteries carry the "good stuff," but in this specific loop, they are the delivery trucks heading to the cleaning station.

Once that blood reaches the lungs, it spreads out into a massive network of tiny vessels called capillaries. These capillaries are so small that red blood cells have to line up and pass through them in single file. These vessels wrap around millions of tiny air sacs called alveoli. This is the great exchange. Through a process called diffusion, the carbon dioxide leaps out of your blood and into your lungs so you can exhale it. At the same moment, the oxygen you just inhaled leaps into your blood. In the blink of an eye, that dull, purple blood turns a brilliant, bright scarlet. It is now "charged" and ready for action. It flows back into the left side of your heart, which then slams it out to the rest of your body with incredible force. This loop happens thousands of times a day, and the efficiency of this exchange determines exactly how much energy you have when you are climbing a flight of stairs or chasing your kids around the yard.

### The Power of Rhythmic Breathing

Now that we know how the system works, how do we make it work better for us? In the world of 90s fitness, we are all about optimization. We don't just want to breathe; we want to breathe with purpose. One of the most common mistakes people make when they start an aerobic program is letting their breathing become erratic. When you gasp for air or take short, shallow sips of breath, you are actually putting more stress on your heart. Your heart senses the lack of steady oxygen and starts beating faster to compensate. This raises your heart rate unnecessarily and makes your workout feel much harder than it actually is. The solution is a technique we call Rhythmic Striding.

Rhythmic Striding is all about synchronization. You want to time your breaths to the rhythm of your feet hitting the pavement. For a moderate power walk, a great starting point is the 3:3 pattern. This means you inhale for three full steps and exhale for three full steps. By doing this, you create a steady, predictable flow of oxygen into the pulmonary loop. Your heart "relaxes" into this rhythm. It knows exactly when the next shipment of oxygen is coming, which allows it to maintain a steady, efficient beat. As you get fitter, you might move to a 4:4 pattern, or if you are pushing into a higher intensity zone, a 2:2 pattern. The specific number matters less than the consistency. When your breath and your stride are in harmony, you become an aerobic machine.

Another key component of this strategy is Diaphragmatic Engagement, or what many call "belly breathing." If you watch a baby sleep, you will see their stomach rise and fall, not their chest. Somewhere along the way to adulthood, many of us became "chest breathers." We use the small muscles in our upper chest and neck to pull in air, which only fills the top portion of our lungs. This is inefficient and triggers a stress response in the body. To help your heart, you need to use your diaphragm—the large, dome-shaped muscle at the base of your lungs. When you breathe into your belly, you expand the lower lobes of your lungs, where the most blood flow occurs. This means you get more "bang for your buck" with every breath. More oxygen enters the blood, and your heart doesn't have to work nearly as hard to keep you fueled.

### Ancient Wisdom: The Concept of Qi

While we have modern science to explain the pulmonary loop, humans have known about the vital connection between breath and energy for thousands of years. If we look back at ancient Chinese medicine, we find the concept of *Qi* (pronounced "chee"). While *Qi* is often translated as "life force" or "energy," it is also deeply synonymous with the word for "breath." The ancients believed that we are born with a certain amount of original energy, but that we must constantly replenish it through the air we breathe and the food we eat.

In this traditional view, the chest was seen as the "Sea of Qi." The heart and lungs were not viewed as two separate organs doing two separate jobs, but as a single functional unit that transformed the air into the energy that moves our limbs and clears our minds. They believed that shallow breathing led to "stagnant Qi," which would eventually manifest as physical weakness or even emotional sadness. To keep the heart healthy, one had to keep the breath flowing. Practices like Tai Chi and Qigong were developed specifically to coordinate slow, deep breathing with deliberate movement. Even though they didn't have microscopes to see capillaries or red blood cells, they arrived at the same conclusion we have today: your vitality is directly linked to the quality of your breath. When you practice your rhythmic breathing during your morning walk, you are participating in a tradition of health that stretches back through the centuries.

### Action Steps for a High-Oxygen Lifestyle

It is time to take these concepts out of the book and into your daily life. You don't need a gym membership to improve your lung-heart connection; you just need a bit of focus and a few minutes of your time. Here is your action plan for the week. These steps are designed to strengthen your respiratory muscles and protect your pulmonary system from outside interference.

1. **The 5-Minute Box Breathing Session:** This is a powerful tool for calming the nervous system and lowering your heart rate. Sit comfortably in a chair with your back straight. You are going to breathe in a "square" or "box" pattern. Inhale slowly through your nose for a count of

four. Hold that breath in for a count of four. Exhale slowly through your mouth for a count of four. Finally, hold your lungs empty for a count of four. Repeat this for five minutes. This exercise trains your diaphragm and teaches your heart to stay calm under the pressure of a controlled breath hold. It is a fantastic way to start your day or wind down before bed.

2. **The Rhythmic Walking Check:** On your next power walk, I want you to spend the first ten minutes focusing entirely on your breath-to-step ratio. Start with the 3:3 pattern (inhale for three steps, exhale for three steps). If you feel like you are gasping, slow your walking pace down until the breathing feels comfortable. Once you find that rhythm, try to maintain it for the rest of your walk. Notice how much more "in control" you feel. By the end of the week, this should start to feel like second nature. You are training your brain to automate a high-performance breathing pattern.

3. **Environmental Awareness:** Your lungs are delicate, and they are the only internal organ constantly exposed to the outside world. Today, make a conscious effort to avoid respiratory irritants. The biggest culprit is second-hand smoke. If you are in a restaurant or a public space, choose the non-smoking section. If you live in an area with high smog, try to do your outdoor exercise in the early morning when the air quality is usually at its best. If you are cleaning the house, make sure the area is well-ventilated so you aren't breathing in harsh chemical fumes. Think of it as protecting the air intake of your high-performance engine. You wouldn't put cheap, dirty gas in a Ferrari, so don't put dirty air in your lungs.

4. **The Lung Capacity Check:** This is a simple way to gauge your respiratory efficiency. Take a deep, full breath until your lungs feel completely expanded. Start a timer and see how long you can steadily exhale through pursed lips (like you are blowing through a straw). A healthy set of lungs should be able to provide a steady stream of air for at least 25 to 30 seconds. If you find yourself running out of air in 10 or 15 seconds, it is a sign that your respiratory muscles need more training. Don't worry—as you continue with your walking program and your box breathing, you will see this number climb.

### Common Pitfalls to Avoid

As you embark on this journey to better heart and lung health, there are a few traps that many people fall into. The first is "Holding the Breath." This often happens when people are lifting something heavy or trying to maintain a difficult pace. This is called the Valsalva maneuver, and it causes a sudden, sharp spike in blood pressure. While it might give you a temporary burst of stability, it puts a massive amount of strain on your heart valves. Always remember: if you are moving, you should be breathing. Never "lock" your breath during exercise.

The second pitfall is ignoring the nose. Your nose is a sophisticated filtration and humidification system. It warms the air and filters out dust and debris before it ever reaches your lungs. Whenever possible, especially during low-to-moderate intensity exercise, try to inhale through your nose. Save the mouth-breathing for those high-intensity bursts when you absolutely need the maximum volume of air. Nose breathing helps maintain the right balance of carbon dioxide in your blood, which actually helps your tissues release oxygen more easily. It is a subtle tweak that makes a big difference in how you feel.

Finally, don't ignore "sticky" lungs. If you find yourself coughing frequently during exercise or feeling an unusual tightness in your chest that doesn't go away when you slow down, don't just push through it. While we want to challenge ourselves, we have to listen to the signals our body is sending. Exercise-induced asthma or simple allergies can hamper your progress. If your "intake" is struggling, your "engine" will suffer. Consult with a professional if your breathing feels like it is hitting a wall that exercise alone won't fix.

**Reflecting on Your Internal Engine**

Take a moment to think about your current habits. When you are stressed at work, do you notice your breath getting shallow and moving up into your chest? This is your body entering "fight or flight" mode, and your heart is paying the price. By becoming aware of these patterns, you can intervene. You have the power to manually override your nervous system just by changing the way you breathe. It is the most direct way to speak to your heart and tell it that everything is okay.

Ask yourself: how can I better support my lungs to help my heart? Maybe it's taking those five minutes for box breathing, or maybe it's finally deciding to stay away from smoky environments for good. Every choice you make to improve your breathing is a direct deposit into your heart health account. You are building a system that is resilient, efficient, and ready for the long haul. The partnership between your heart and lungs is the foundation of your physical existence. When they work together in harmony, there is no limit to the vitality you can achieve.

We have spent this time looking at the engine and the intake. We've seen how they are linked by the pulmonary loop and how we can use rhythmic breathing to make the whole system run smoother. We've even looked back at ancient cultures who understood these truths long before we had modern medical imaging. You now have a practical set of tools to ensure that your heart is getting the high-quality oxygen it needs to beat strong and steady. This is what it means to take ownership of your health. You aren't just a passenger in your body; you are the lead mechanic, the driver, and the navigator all rolled into one.

As you move forward into the next week, pay attention to the air around you. Feel the expansion of your ribs and the steady beat of your heart. You are a biological masterpiece of engineering, and you are finally learning how to handle the controls. Keep practicing that 3:3 stride, keep breathing deep into your belly, and keep protecting your internal environment. Your heart is counting on your lungs, and your lungs are counting on you. It's a team effort, and so far, you are doing a great job leading the way. Stay focused, stay rhythmic, and keep moving toward that goal of a stronger, more vibrant you.

The journey of heart health is a marathon, not a sprint. It is built on the small, daily decisions to breathe a little deeper and move a little more intentionally. You have already taken the most important steps by educating yourself and committing to a plan. As we continue, we will explore even more ways to refine your "engine" and clear the "highways" of your body. But for now, just breathe. Feel the oxygen entering your blood, turning it bright red, and fueling the very muscle that keeps you alive. It is a beautiful, constant cycle of renewal. Treasure it, train it, and watch as your energy levels soar to heights you haven't felt in years. You are well on your way to mastering your own vitality, one breath at a time.

# Chapter 4
## Blood Vessels:
## The Superhighways of Health

Think about the last time you were stuck in a massive traffic jam on the highway. You were probably sitting there, gripped by frustration, watching the minutes tick away while the cars ahead of you remained motionless. The engine was humming, the fuel was ready to burn, but you weren't going anywhere because the road itself was blocked. This is exactly how your body feels when your circulation is sluggish. You can have the strongest cardiac muscle in the world, but that strength is wasted if the delivery system is falling apart. Your blood vessels are the superhighways of your health, stretching over 60,000 miles if you were to lay them out end to end. That is enough to circle the globe twice! If these roads are cracked, narrowed, or lose their ability to expand, your vitality comes to a screeching halt. To live a long, energetic life, you have to care for the pipes as much as the pump.

Your blood vessels are not just passive tubes; they are dynamic, living tissues that respond to every move you make and every glass of water you drink. They possess a quality that is perhaps the truest indicator of youth: elasticity. When your vessels are supple and flexible, they can handle the surges of pressure that come with a brisk walk or a stressful day at the office. When they become stiff and brittle Your circulatory system is divided into three main types of vessels, each with a specific job to do. If you think of your body as a city, the **arteries** are the major interstates. These are the thick-walled, muscular tubes that carry oxygenated blood away from the heart. Because they are receiving blood directly from the heart's powerful left ventricle, they are under high pressure. This is why their walls are so thick. They need to be able to stretch when the heart beats and snap back into place when the heart rests. This "snap" actually helps push the blood along, acting like a secondary pump. When an artery loses that snap, we call it hardening, and it is a major contributor to high blood pressure.

At the other end of the journey, we have the **veins**. Think of these as the return lanes heading back to the city center. Once the blood has delivered its oxygen and nutrients, it has to get back to the heart to be recharged. However, there is a catch: the pressure in the veins is very low. By the time blood reaches your feet and starts the long climb back up to your chest, it has lost almost all the momentum it got from the heart. To fight gravity, your veins are equipped with one-way valves. These valves act like tiny locks in a canal, allowing blood to move up but preventing it from flowing backward. This is also why movement is so vital for vein health. Your leg muscles act as a manual pump, squeezing the veins and forcing the blood upward. If you sit still for hours, that blood pools in your ankles, which is why your shoes might feel tight at the end of a long flight or a sedentary workday.

Finally, we have the **capillaries**. These are the local streets and alleys where the actual business of life happens. They are so small that they are only one cell thick—so thin that red blood cells literally have to squeeze through them in single file. This thinness is intentional. It allows oxygen, sugar, and hormones to pass through the vessel walls and into your tissues, while waste products like carbon dioxide move in the opposite direction.

While they might be small, they are incredibly numerous. Almost every cell in your body is within a hair's breadth of a capillary. When your circulation is healthy, this "micro-circulation" is efficient and fast. When it is poor, your cells start to starve and accumulate waste, leaving you feeling sluggish and tired.

### The Science of Elasticity and Pressure

The term **blood pressure** is something we hear all the time, but what does it actually mean for your vessels? Imagine a garden hose. If the hose is wide and flexible, the water flows through easily even if you turn the faucet up high. But if the hose is narrow or made of stiff, unyielding plastic, the pressure inside skyrockets. In your body, blood pressure is a measurement of the force your blood exerts against the walls of your arteries. It is expressed in two numbers: systolic and diastolic. The systolic number (the top one) is the pressure when your heart is actively beating. The diastolic number (the bottom one) is the pressure in the vessels when your heart is resting between beats.

The key to a healthy reading is the **elasticity** of the arterial walls. When your heart pumps, level. As you age, or if you eat a diet high in saturated fats and refined sugars, those walls can become stiff. When the heart pumps blood into a stiff, narrow tube, the pressure spikes. Over time, this high pressure causes microscopic tears in the vessel lining. Your body tries to patch these tears with a combination of cholesterol and minerals, creating what we know as plaque. This plaque further narrows the vessel, causing the pressure to rise even more. It is a dangerous cycle that can lead to serious complications, but the good news is that lifestyle changes can help maintain and even restore much of that vital flexibility.

## The Vessel Flush: Your Daily Circulation Strategy

In our modern world, we spend far too much time being stationary. Whether it is sitting in front of a computer, driving in a car, or relaxing on the sofa, our bodies are often in a state of "circulatory stagnation." To combat this, we use a simple but effective approach called the **Vessel Flush**. This isn't a fancy supplement or a complicated medical procedure; it is a two-pronged strategy involving hydration and strategic movement designed to keep your blood moving and your vessel walls healthy.

The first part of the flush is When you are dehydrated, your blood becomes thicker and more viscous—think of it like trying to pump cold molasses through a straw instead of water. Thick blood requires more pressure to move, which puts extra strain on your heart and your vessel walls. By enough to glide through those tiny capillaries without resistance. Many people reach for coffee or caffeinated sodas when they feel tired, but these can actually act as diuretics, pulling water out of your system. If you want a real energy boost, try a large glass of pure water first. It thins the blood and speeds up the delivery of oxygen to your brain and muscles.

The second part of the flush involves Low-Impact Movement. As we discussed, your veins need help getting blood back to the heart. The most effective way to provide this help is by using your "second heart"—the calf muscles. Every time you flex your calves, they compress the deep veins in your legs, shooting blood upward toward your torso. This is why long periods of sitting are so draining. Without that muscular pump, your circulation slows down, and your heart has to work harder to overcome the lack of return flow. By incorporating short, frequent bursts of movement into your day, you "flush" the system, preventing blood from pooling and ensuring a fresh supply of oxygenated blood reaches every corner is easy to take our knowledge of blood vessels for granted, but for most of human history, the internal workings of the "pipes" were a complete mystery. In the early 1900s, medical science underwent a massive shift in how it viewed the aging process. Before this era, it was generally assumed that becoming frail and weak was simply an inevitable part of getting older—something that happened to everyone, like gray hair or wrinkled skin. However, as doctors began performing more detailed autopsies, they noticed a recurring pattern in people who had suffered from "old age" ailments.

Researchers found that the arteries of these individuals weren't soft and pliable like those of a young person. Instead, they were often hard, crunchy, and filled with yellowish deposits. They called this condition arteriosclerosis, or "hardening of the arteries." This discovery was a turning point because it suggested that many of the symptoms we associated with aging were actually the result of a specific physical breakdown in the circulatory system. If the vessels were the problem, then perhaps there were ways to protect them. This realization gave birth to the modern field of preventative medicine. We began to understand that a man is only as old as his arteries. If you keep your vessels clean and elastic, you can maintain the vigor of a much younger person well into your later years. This 90s era of fitness is the culmination of that research, giving you the tools to fight back against the "hardening" that previous generations thought was unavoidable.

## Your Practical Action Plan

It is time to put this knowledge into motion. You don't need expensive equipment to improve your vascular health; you just need consistency and awareness. These three steps are designed to be integrated into your normal routine, starting today. By focusing on these habits, you are actively protecting the elasticity of your vessels and ensuring your "superhighways" stay open for business.

1. **The 8-Glass Hydration Challenge:** Today, your primary goal is to consume at least eight 8-ounce glasses of water. To make this easier, carry a dedicated water bottle with you. Drink one glass immediately upon waking up to rehydrate your system after a night of sleep. Then, have another glass before every meal. Not only does this help your blood volume, but it also aids in digestion and can help with weight management. If you find plain water boring, add a slice of lemon or lime, but avoid the sugary "fruit drinks" that are often loaded with high-fructose corn syrup. Your vessels want pure H2O to keep that blood flowing smoothly.

2. **The Hourly Circulation Break:** Set a timer on your watch or computer for every 60 minutes. When it goes off, I want you to spend just two minutes moving your legs. If you can get up and walk around the office, great! If you are stuck in a meeting or on a phone call, you can perform Calve Pump Exercises while seated. Simply lift your heels as high as they can go while keeping your toes on the floor, hold for a second, and then lower them. Do this 20 to 30 times. This simple action engages the calf-

vein pump and prevents the "heavy leg" feeling that comes from sitting too long. It is a quick way to refresh your energy levels without even leaving your desk.

3. **Know Your Numbers:** You cannot manage what you do not measure. Schedule a visit to your local pharmacy or your doctor's office this week to get a professional blood pressure reading. Many grocery stores now have automated machines that are free to use. Write down your numbers. A healthy reading is typically around 120/80. If your numbers are consistently higher than 140/90, it is a signal that your vessels are under too much stress. Don't be afraid of the data; use it as a baseline. As you improve your diet and stick to your walking routine, you will have the immense satisfaction of watching those numbers drop into the healthy zone.

## Common Mistakes to Watch For

One of the most dangerous misconceptions people have is thinking that high blood pressure—often called the "silent killer"—will have obvious symptoms. Many folks believe they will feel a headache or a sense of "pounding" in their chest if their pressure is high. The reality is that you can feel perfectly fine while your arteries are being damaged by excessive force. This is why regular monitoring is non-negotiable. Don't wait for a sign; go get checked.

Another frequent error is the "weekend warrior" approach to movement. Some people sit all week and then try to make up for it with a grueling three-hour hike on Sunday. While the hike is good, it doesn't undo the damage of five days of stagnation. Your blood vessels thrive on frequent, moderate movement. It is far better for your circulation to take five 10-minute walks throughout the day than to do one long session and remain motionless for the rest of the time. Think of it like a stream; a steady flow keeps the water clear, while a stagnant pond becomes murky, even if you throw a bucket of fresh water in it once a week.

Finally, be wary of “liquid energy.” We live in a fast-paced world, and it is tempting to rely on caffeinated sodas and energy drinks to get through the day. While these might give you a temporary lift, they are often double-trouble for your vessels. The caffeine can cause temporary constriction of the arteries, raising your blood pressure, while the high sugar content can lead to inflammation in the vessel lining. If you are and Awareness

Take a moment to evaluate your current daily rhythm. Do you spend more than four hours a day sitting down? If so, your vessels are likely crying out for a “flush.” Think about how your legs feel at 5:00 PM. Are they swollen? Do they feel heavy or restless? These are the early warning signs of sluggish circulation. By becoming mindful of these physical cues, you can take action before minor discomfort turns into a chronic issue.

Ask yourself: Is my hydration supporting my blood volume? If you only drink when you are already parched, you are already behind the curve. Dehydration is a stressor that your heart has to compensate for every single minute. By making water your beverage of choice, you are providing the very foundation of cardiovascular health. It is a simple habit, but its impact on your long-term vitality is massive.

Remember, your blood vessels are the life-giving network that sustains every organ, every muscle, and every thought. When they are healthy, you feel light, energetic, and sharp. When they are neglected, everything becomes a struggle. You have the power to keep these superhighways open and clear. Through the simple acts of drinking water, moving your legs, and monitoring your pressure, you are taking ownership of your circulatory destiny. You aren't just preventing disease; you are building a foundation for a high-performance life. Keep those pipes clean, keep that blood moving, and you will feel the difference in every step you take. Your heart works hard for you; the least you can do is give it a smooth road to run on.

As we move forward, we will continue to build on this foundation. We have explored the engine, the intake, and now the highways. Each piece of the puzzle fits together to create a stronger, more resilient version of you. The journey to heart health is not about radical, overnight changes; it is about these small, smart choices that add up over time. Stay consistent with your hydration, keep those circulation breaks on your schedule, and always keep an eye on your numbers. You are doing the work that pays off in decades of health and vitality. Let's keep that momentum going as we dive deeper into the lifestyle habits that will make your heart—and your vessels—invincible.

# Chapter 5
## Muscles and the Heart: The Strength Connection

Have you ever considered that your skeletal muscles might be the most underrated assistants your cardiovascular system has? Most people look at a pair of dumbbells and think about building bigger biceps for the beach, or they see someone doing squats and imagine a bodybuilder preparing for a competition. But there is a much more functional reason to care about your muscle tone, and it has everything to do with that tireless pump in your chest. When you strengthen your body, you aren't just changing how you look in a mirror; you are fundamentally altering the physics of how your blood moves. Stronger muscles create a more efficient environment for your heart, allowing it to do more work with less effort. If you want to live a long, vibrant life, you need to start thinking of your muscles as the secondary engines of your circulatory system.

The relationship between your heart and your muscles is a two-way street. We often talk about how the heart pumps blood to the muscles to give them energy, but we rarely discuss the reverse. Your muscles actually help the heart by facilitating the return of blood and by reducing the resistance the heart has to pump against. Think of it like a team of rowers in a boat. The heart is the coxswain, setting the pace and providing the primary force, but if the rowers—your muscles—are weak and sluggish, the boat barely moves despite the coxswain's best efforts. When those rowers are strong and coordinated system in a whole new light: as a vital partner in your quest for peak cardiac health.

### Anatomy 101: The Pump Behind the Pump

To understand why strength training is a cardiac necessity, we have to talk about a concept called peripheral resistance. This is a term doctors use to describe the opposition to blood flow within the systemic circulation. Imagine your heart is a water pump trying to push liquid through a series of tubes. If those tubes are narrow or if there is nothing helping the fluid along at the far ends of the system, the pump has to work much harder to maintain the flow. In your body, the "far ends" are your arms and legs. When your muscles are toned and active, they act as a physiological squeeze that assists the veins in moving blood back toward the center of your body. This is often called the **skeletal muscle pump**.

Every time a muscle contracts, it compresses the nearby veins. Because your veins have one-way valves, this compression forces the blood to move in only one direction: back toward the heart. If your muscles are weak or underused, this return flow becomes sluggish. The blood pools in the lower extremities, and the heart has to exert more pressure to keep things moving. This extra pressure translates to a higher heart rate and more wear and tear on your arterial walls. By maintaining a baseline of muscular strength, you are essentially installing a series of booster pumps throughout your body. This reduces the workload on your heart, lowering your resting heart rate and helping to keep your blood pressure in stress it feels at the core.

Furthermore, muscle tissue is metabolically active in a way that fat is not. Even when you are sitting on the couch watching the evening news, your muscles are burning calories and processing oxygen. Having a higher ratio of muscle to fat improves your body's insulin sensitivity and its ability to manage blood sugar. High blood sugar is a major irritant to the lining of your blood vessels, leading to the buildup of plaque. Therefore, by building muscle, you are creating a chemical environment that protects your heart. You aren't just building a stronger frame; you are building a more resilient chemical processing plant that keeps your blood clean and your vessels flexible. This is why resistance training is just as important as your morning walk or your afternoon jog.

### The 90s Approach: Light Resistance for Heavy Results

In the current fitness climate, we are seeing a shift away from the "bulking up" mentality of previous decades. We now understand that you don't need to look like a professional wrestler to reap the benefits of strength training. In fact, for heart health, the most effective method is often **Light Resistance Training**. This involves using relatively low weights—think endurance and tone rather than pure mass, which is exactly what your heart needs to stay healthy. It improves the quality of the muscle fiber and the density of the capillaries within those muscles, providing more channels for blood to flow through.

Keep blood circulating throughout the entire body during your workout. Instead of doing three sets of bicep curls and then resting the exercises alternate between the upper and lower body, your heart has to work to shunt blood from one extremity to the other. This prevents blood from pooling in one specific area and forces the circulatory system to remain highly active. It is a fantastic way to get a cardiovascular workout while simultaneously toning your muscles. It turns your strength routine into a heart-pumping circuit that builds stamina and strength all at once.

Bodyweight calisthenics are another pillar of this heart-smart strategy. Exercises like push-ups, squats, and planks are incredible because they require multiple muscle groups to work in harmony. This "compound" movement mimics the way we move in real life—lifting groceries, climbing stairs, or picking up a grandchild. When you train your muscles to work together, you improve your functional fitness, which makes daily tasks less taxing on your heart. If your legs are strong, walking up a flight of stairs doesn't send your heart rate into19th century, the "Strongman" was a popular figure in circuses and traveling shows. Men like Eugen Sandow became famous for their incredible physiques and feats of strength, such as lifting horses or breaking chains. During this era, strength was seen as a spectacle, a freakish display of power that had little to do with the health of the average person. In fact, many people at the time believed that "heavy" exercise could actually damage the heart, leading to a condition they called "athletic heart," which they feared would cause an early death. They saw the heart as a delicate organ that should be protected from the strain of heavy lifting.

However, as we moved into the 20th century, medical science began to debunk these myths. We started to realize that the heart, being a muscle itself, actually thrives on the right kind of challenge. By the middle of the century, researchers began to link sedentary lifestyles with a rise in heart disease. The focus shifted from the "spectacle" of strength to the "utility" of strength. We began to understand that the human body was designed for movement and resistance. The evolution of fitness moved away from the extreme lifting of the strongmen toward the balanced, functional fitness we advocate for today. We now know that a moderate amount of muscle tone is one of the best predictors of longevity.

Today, we view the body as a holistic system. We no longer separate "cardio" from "strength" as if they were two unrelated goals. We recognize that they are two sides of the same coin. The strength of your legs supports the health of your heart, and the health of your heart allows you to maintain the strength of your legs. This shift in perspective has allowed us to develop routines that are accessible to everyone, regardless of age or starting fitness level. You don't have to be a 19th-century strongman to have a heart that is strong enough to last for ninety years. You just need to give your muscles enough work to keep them active and engaged in the process of living.

### Common Pitfalls in Strength Training

While adding resistance to your routine is vital, there are a few common mistakes that can actually put unnecessary stress on your heart. The first is the habit of holding your breath during a lift. This is sudden, sharp increase in internal thoracic pressure, which can cause a rapid spike in blood pressure and then a sudden drop. should exhale during the most difficult part of the movement (the "work" phase) and inhale as you return to the starting

Another frequent error is focusing exclusively on the "mirror muscles"—the chest and biceps—while ignoring the lower body. This is a mistake for two reasons. First, your leg muscles (the glutes, quads, and ham skeletal muscle pump and your overall metabolic rate. Training your legs provides the biggest "bang for your buck" when it comes to assisting your heart. Second, an unbalanced body is an inefficient body. If your upper body is heavy and your legs are weak, your heart has to work harder to move that weight around. A heart-healthy routine should always be full-body, ensuring that every part of the "secondary pump" system is operational.

Finally, avoid the trap of "too much, too soon." Many people get motivated to start a new routine and immediately reach for the heaviest weights they can find. This often leads to poor form, which results in joint pain or muscle strains that sideline you for weeks. For the sake of your heart, consistency lift a heavy weight three times with bad form. Your goal isn't to set a world record; it's to create a steady, rhythmic contraction that helps your blood flow. If you feel like you are straining to the point of turning red in the face, you are likely working against your heart rather than with it. Lighten the load and focus on the rhythm of your movement and breath.

### Your Resistance Action Plan

It is time to start building that secondary pump. You don't need a gym membership or a room full of expensive machines to get started. These By following this plan, you will begin to feel the difference in your energy levels and your overall stamina within just a few weeks.

1. **The 10-Squat Heart Test:** This is a simple way to see how your muscles and heart interact. Stand with your feet shoulder-width apart. Slowly lower your hips as if you are sitting back into an invisible chair, keeping your chest up

and your weight on your heels. Perform 10 controlled squats. Notice how your heart rate begins to rise. This isn't just because your heart is working harder; it's because your large leg muscles are demanding more oxygen and are simultaneously pushing blood back up to your chest. If you feel winded after just ten, that is a sign that your "rowers" need more training. Incorporate these into your day—do ten while waiting for the coffee to brew or during a commercial break on TV.

2. **Identify Your Major Muscle Groups:** To build an effective routine, you need to know which muscles you are targeting. For heart health, you want to focus on the "big five": the legs, the back, the chest, the shoulders, and the core. Write down one simple exercise for each. For example: Squats (legs), Wall Push-ups (chest and shoulders), Bird-Dogs (back and core). By having a plan for each major area, you ensure that your entire circulatory system is getting the support it needs. You don't have to do them all at once; you can rotate through them throughout the day to keep your blood moving.

3. **The Hand Weight Investment:** Go out and purchase a set of light hand weights, preferably in the three-to-five-pound range. If you don't want to buy weights, you can use two full water bottles or even two cans of soup from your pantry. Having these physical objects serves as a visual reminder to do your "toning" work. Once or twice a day, pick them up and do a few minutes of bicep curls, lateral raises, or overhead presses. These small bouts of resistance keep the muscles in your arms and shoulders firm, preventing blood from stagnating in the upper

extremities and helping the heart maintain a smooth, steady flow.

### Reflecting on Strength

As you begin this journey, take a moment to ask yourself: have you been avoiding weights because you fear "bulking up" or looking like a bodybuilder? It is a common misconception, especially for women or older adults. But remember, muscle is the armor of your heart. Without it, your heart is forced to do all the heavy lifting on its own. How can strength serve your heart today? Perhaps it means being able to carry the groceries in one trip without feeling out of breath. Perhaps it means having the stability to walk on an uneven trail with confidence. When you view strength through the lens of heart health, it ceases to be about vanity and becomes about **vitality**.

Your heart is a remarkable organ, but it was never meant to work in isolation. It is part of a grand, integrated system that relies on the health of your vessels, the capacity of your lungs, and the strength of your muscles. By toning your body, you are giving your heart the gift of efficiency. You are making every beat count for more. You are ensuring that your circulation is active and vibrant from the tips of your fingers to the soles of your feet. This is the essence of heart-smart living: recognizing that every part of you belongs to the whole, and every part of you has a role to play in keeping the engine running.

Keep focused on the feeling of your muscles working. Feel the squeeze in your calves, the tension in your core, and the power in your legs. These sensations are the signs that your secondary pumps are online and doing their job. As you continue to build this foundation, you will find that you have more energy, less fatigue, and a greater sense of control over your physical well-being. Your heart is the leader, but your muscles are the dedicated crew that makes the journey possible. Give them the attention they deserve, and they will reward you with a lifetime of steady, reliable performance. We are building a body that is not just strong on the outside, but resilient and efficient on the inside. Let's keep moving toward that goal, one rep and one heartbeat at a time.

In the next phase of our journey, we will look at how the nervous system acts as the command center for this entire operation. Your heart doesn't just beat on its own; it follows a complex set of signals from your brain and nerves. Understanding how to manage those signals through relaxation and stress control is the final piece of the cardiovascular puzzle. But for now, focus on your strength. Pick up those light weights, do those squats, and feel the incredible power of a body that works in perfect harmony. You are doing the work that matters, and your heart is feeling the benefit of every single movement you make.

# Chapter 6
## The Nervous System:
## The Heart's Command Center

Imagine your body is a high-performance sports car. You have the engine, which is that magnificent pump in your chest, and the fuel, which is the nutrition you eat. But what about the electrical system? What about the wires and the computer chips that tell the engine when to rev up and when to idle? That role belongs to your nervous system. It is the silent director behind the scenes, making split-second decisions that determine whether your pulse stays steady or starts racing like a runaway train. If you have ever felt your heart leap into your throat when a car suddenly swerves into your lane, you have experienced the power of this system firsthand. It is fast, it is precise, and it is completely in control of how your cardiovascular system reacts to the world around you.

Most of us go through our day thinking of our emotions as something that happens only in our heads. We feel "stressed" or "anxious" as if these are purely mental states. But your heart knows better. To your heart, every thought is a physical command. The brain does not keep its worries to itself; it broadcasts them through a network of nerves that wrap around your heart like a set of reins. When those reins are pulled tight, your heart responds instantly. If you want to master your health, you have to learn how to talk back to your brain. You need to understand the language of the nervous system so you can tell your heart to settle down when the world gets too loud.

## The Hidden Wiring: Anatomy 101

To get a handle on this, we need to look at the Autonomic Nervous System, or the ANS. This is the part of your wiring that handles everything you do not have to think about. It manages your digestion, your breathing, and most importantly, your heart rate. The ANS is divided into two main branches that act like a gas pedal and a brake. They are always in a tug-of-war, trying to keep your body in a state of perfect balance. When one side wins out for too long, that is when you start to see problems with your blood pressure and your overall energy levels.

The first branch is the **Sympathetic Nervous System**. This is your "Fight or Flight" response. It is an ancient survival mechanism that evolved to help our ancestors escape from predators or defend their territory. When the Sympathetic system kicks in, it floods your body with hormones like adrenaline. This causes your heart to beat faster and harder so it can pump more blood to your large muscles. Your pupils dilate, your breathing becomes shallow, and your body shuts down non-essential functions like digestion. In short bursts, this is a life-saver. It gives you the edge you need to handle a genuine emergency. However, in our modern world, the Sympathetic system often gets stuck in the "on" position. Your body cannot tell the difference between a mountain lion and a missed deadline at work. If you are constantly in this state, your heart is being forced to run at a high RPM for no good reason, which leads to exhaustion and wear.

The second branch is the **Parasympathetic Nervous System**. This is the "Rest and Digest" side of the house. This is your body's natural braking system. When the Parasympathetic system is in charge, your heart rate slows down, your blood pressure drops, and your body focuses on repair and recovery. This is the state where your heart gets to rest. It is the time when your cells are rejuvenated and your energy stores are replenished. The goal of a heart-healthy lifestyle is to ensure that the Parasympathetic system gets plenty of "airtime." Unfortunately, many of us have forgotten how to activate this brake. We live in a society that prizes being busy and "on the go," which means we are effectively driving our cars with our feet slammed down on the gas pedal twenty-four hours a day.

The communication between these two systems and your heart is a two-way street. It is not just that the brain tells the heart what to do; the heart also sends signals back to the brain. When your heart rate is high and irregular, it sends messages to the brain that say, "We are in danger!" This creates a feedback loop of anxiety. By learning to control your physical state, you can actually change your mental state. You can use your body to calm your mind, which in turn calms your heart. It is a powerful realization: you are not just a victim of your nerves. You are the operator of the system.

### The 90s Wellness Strategy: Autogenic Visualization

Since we know that the brain and heart are in a constant conversation, we can use that to our advantage. Back in the early 1990s, a technique called **Autogenic Visualization** became a staple of high-performance stress management. It is a way of using specific mental images to trigger a physical response in the body. Instead of just "trying to relax," which almost never works when you are actually stressed, you give your brain a specific set of instructions that the Parasympathetic system understands. This is like a "manual override" for your heart rate.

Another powerful tool is the "Ocean Breath" visualization. Close your eyes and imagine the rhythm of the tide coming in and going out on a quiet beach. Synchronize your breathing with this image. As the wave rolls onto the sand, take a slow, deep breath in through your nose. As the wave recedes back into the ocean, let your breath out slowly through your mouth. Do not force it; just let it flow. By linking your breath to a steady, natural rhythm, you are sending a clear signal to your Autonomic Nervous System that the "emergency" is over. Within sixty seconds, you will likely find that your pulse has dropped by several beats per minute. This is not magic; it is biology. You are using the visual centers of your brain to pull the Parasympathetic brake.

These techniques are most effective when they are practiced regularly, not just when you are in the middle of a crisis. Think of it like training a muscle. You want to build the "relaxation response" so that it is ready to go whenever you need it. If you spend five minutes every morning doing these visualizations, your body becomes more efficient at switching from the Sympathetic to the Parasympathetic state. You are essentially teaching your heart how to recover more quickly. In the high-stress world of the 90s, this was the secret weapon of corporate executives and elite athletes alike. It is about taking the wheel and refusing to let your circumstances dictate your physical well-being.

## The Heart Through Time: From Hysteria to Stress

It is fascinating to look back at how we have understood the link between the nerves and the heart over the centuries. In the Victorian era, doctors were obsessed with conditions they called "Hysteria" or "Nervous Exhaustion" (also known as Neurasthenia). They believed that the nervous system had a limited amount of "nerve force" or energy. If a person worked too hard, thought too much, or experienced too much emotional turmoil, they would "leak" this energy until they became physically ill. The symptoms were often cardiovascular: palpitations, a racing pulse, and chest pains. The prescribed cure back then was often the "Rest Cure," where patients—mostly women—were forced to stay in bed for weeks in total silence and isolation.

While the Victorians were wrong about "nerve force" being a finite fluid, they were right about the fact that the nervous system can be overwhelmed. They saw the physical impact of a life that was moving too fast. As the Industrial Revolution picked up speed, people were suddenly exposed to more noise, more light, and more social pressure than ever before. Their hearts were reacting to the "modern" pace of life. However people were simply too "sensitive" for the world they had built.

Fast forward to the middle of the 20th century, and the conversation shifted toward "Stress." This term was popularized by Hans Selye, a researcher who realized that the body has a non-specific response to any demand made upon it. Whether you are freezing cold, because it moved the focus away from "nerves" as a sign of weakness and toward "stress" as a physiological event. We began to realize that the heart was the primary target of this response. The "Type A" personality became a household to heart attacks because their Sympathetic systems never turned off.

Today, we have more data than the Victorians could have ever dreamed of, but we are facing the same basic problem. We are living in a world that is designed to keep us in a state of high alert. The constant "ping" of notifications and the twenty-four-hour news cycle are the modern versions of the steam engine and the telegraph. The difference is that we now have the tools to manage it. We know that "nervous exhaustion" is really just the Autonomic Nervous System being pushed past its limits. We do not need a three-month "Rest Cure" in a sanitarium; we need daily habits that activate the Parasympathetic system and protect the heart from the corrosive effects of chronic adrenaline.

## Common Mistakes: The Caffeine and Anxiety Trap

One of the biggest hurdles to a calm heart is how we choose to "self-medicate" our fatigue. When we feel the "nervous exhaustion" the Victorians talked about, our first instinct is usually to reach for another cup of coffee or a caffeinated soda. We think we are tired, so we need a boost. But if your fatigue is caused by a Sympathetic system that is already overworked, adding caffeine is like throwing gasoline on a fire. Caffeine mimics the effects of adrenaline. It binds to the receptors in your heart and tells it to beat faster. If you are already stressed, that extra caffeine can push you into a state of "the jitters," where your heart rate stays elevated even when you are trying to relax.

Another common mistake is ignoring the physical signs of anxiety. Many people think that because they do not "feel" worried in their head, they must not be stressed. But the body often registers stress long before the conscious mind does. If you notice that you are clenching your jaw, that mode. Your heart is already feeling the impact. If you wait until you feel "stressed out" to do something about it, you have already allowed your heart to endure minutes or hours of unnecessary strain. You have to learn to read your body's early warning signals.

We also tend to fall into the trap of thinking that stress is "all in our head." We tell ourselves to "just get over it" or "stop worrying." This is a mistake because it ignores the physical reality of the situation. Stress is a chemical event. Once the adrenaline is in your bloodstream, you cannot just "think" it away. You have to physically process it. This is why techniques like deep breathing and visualization are so important. They provide a physical counter be much more successful at protecting your heart.

Lastly, do not underestimate the impact of "micro-stressors." These are the small things—a messy desk, a flickering light, a loud television in the background—that keep your nervous system on edge. Individually, they are nothing. But collectively, they keep your Sympathetic system humming at a low level all day long. This "background noise" prevents your heart from ever reaching a truly restful state. Part of managing your heart health is creating an environment that allows your nervous system to feel safe. If your home or workspace is a constant source of irritation, your heart is paying the price every single day.

## Your Action Plan for a Calm Heart

It is time to take control of your nervous system. These three steps are designed to help you map your triggers and build a more resilient heart. By being proactive, you can ensure that your "gas pedal" and your "brake" are working in harmony.

### Step 1: Identify Your Top Three Stress Triggers

For the next three days, I want you to pay close attention to when your heart starts to race or your chest feels tight. Carry a small notebook or a piece of paper in your pocket. When you feel that surge of "nervous energy," write down what was happening. Was it a specific person? A certain time of day? A particular task? Most of us have "Top Three" triggers that account for the majority of our daily stress. Once you identify them, you can prepare for them. If you know that the afternoon commute always makes your pulse climb, you can go into it with a plan to use your visualization techniques. You are no longer being blindsided by your own biology.

### Step 2: Practice the 'Silent Minute'

This is one of the simplest and most effective ways to reset your nervous system. At least twice a day— minute, sit in total silence. Do not check your phone. Do not listen to the radio. Do not even pray or meditate in the traditional sense. Just sit and be still. Focus on the sensation of your feet on the floor and the air moving in and out of your lungs. This "Silent Minute" acts as a circuit breaker for your Sympathetic system. It gives your heart a brief window of total peace, allowing your blood pressure to stabilize and your brain to "reset" its threat-detection levels.

### Step 3: Audit Your Caffeine Consumption

I want you to take an honest look at how much caffeine you are putting into your system. For one week, keep track of every cup of coffee, tea, or soda you drink. Notice if there is a correlation between your caffeine intake and your feelings of "the jitters" or a racing heart. If you find that your heart rate is consistently high in the afternoons, try cutting out that second or third cup of coffee. Replace it with a glass of water or a herbal tea. Remember, we want your heart to beat because it needs to, not because it is being artificially stimulated by a chemical. You might be surprised at how much calmer your heart feels when you stop forcing it to run on high-octane fuel all day long.

### Reflection and Moving Forward

Take a second to think: when was the last time you felt truly, deeply relaxed? Not just "not working," but a state where your body felt heavy, your mind felt still, and your heart felt like it was resting in a calm pool of water. For many of us, that feeling is a distant memory. We have become so used to the "background hum" of stress that we have forgotten what true peace feels like. But that peace is the natural state of your heart. It is the state where your heart is most efficient and most resilient. It is the foundation of a long and healthy life.

Does your heart race for no physical reason? Do you find yourself checking your pulse and wondering why it is so high when you are just sitting at your desk? These are messages from your nervous system. They are not things to be feared; they are things to be understood. Your heart is telling you that the "gas pedal" has been held down for too long. By using the techniques we have discussed—the visualizations, the silent minutes, and the caffeine audits—you are taking back the reins. You are showing your body that you are the one in charge, not your worries or your schedule.

The brain is a powerful organ, but it can be a bit of a drama queen. It sees a problem and screams "Emergency!" through the nerves. Your job is to be the calm adult in the room. You have to look at the situation and say, "No, this is just a busy day, not a life-threatening crisis." When you do that, your heart believes you. It settles back into a steady, reliable rhythm. This connection between the mind and the heart is one of the most beautiful aspects of human biology. It means that you have the internal tools to protect yourself from the pressures of the outside world.

As you go through your week, remember that every breath is a chance to reset. Every moment of silence is a gift to your cardiovascular system. You are building a life where your heart is not just a muscle that pumps blood, but a partner in your overall well-being. You are learning to listen to its signals and respond with care. This is what it means to truly own your health. You aren't just reacting to life; you are directing it. Your heart is the engine, your nerves are the wires, and you are the driver. Keep your hands on the wheel, keep your eyes on the road, and remember to use the brakes when you need them. A calm heart is a strong heart, and a strong heart is the "Fight or Flight" response to the ancient history of nervous exhaustion. You now have a toolkit for managing the invisible forces that impact your heart every day. Use these tools with confidence. You are not just trying to live longer; you are trying to live better, a steady one. And let it be a reminder that you have everything you need to thrive in this fast-paced world. next discussion, we will shift our focus to the chemistry of the blood itself. We will look at cholesterol—the "stuff" that can either clear the way for your heart or clog up the works. It is a topic that has been surrounded by a lot of myths and confusion, but we are going to break it down into simple, actionable steps. But for now, take a deep breath. Feel your heart beat. And enjoy the calm that comes from knowing you are in control. You are doing the work that matters, and your heart is thanking you for every single second of peace you give it.

# Chapter 7
## Cholesterol:
## Clearing the Path to Longevity

Listen, we need to have a serious talk about the most misunderstood substance in the American diet. It has been the villain of every health magazine, the boogeyman in every doctor's office, and the primary reason you probably feel guilty every time you look at a steak or a wedge of cheese. I am talking about cholesterol. Now, before you start tossing everything in your refrigerator into the trash, you should know that this waxy, fat-like substance is not just some poison lurking in your bloodstream. In fact, your body actually needs it. Your liver produces it every single day to build cell membranes, manufacture hormones like estrogen and testosterone, and produce the bile acids that help you digest fat. The problem is not that cholesterol exists; the problem is when the balance gets out of whack and the "superhighways" of your circulatory system start getting backed up with traffic.

If you imagine your arteries as a series of clear, flexible tubes that carry life-giving blood to every corner of your body, cholesterol is the material that can either keep those tubes maintained or turn them into a clogged mess. When people talk about "high cholesterol," they are usually worried about the stuff sticking to the walls of those tubes, narrowing the path and forcing the pump in your chest to work at a much higher pressure just to get the job done. But did you know that not all the little particles floating in your blood are trying to cause a pile-up?

Some of them are actually the clean-up crew. Understanding who the players are is the first step toward taking ownership of your longevity. You cannot win the game if you do not know which team is which.

## Anatomy 101: Meet the HDL and LDL Teams

To really get a grip on what is happening inside your vessels, you have to understand that cholesterol cannot travel through your blood on its own. Since it is a fat and your blood is mostly water, they do not mix—just like oil and vinegar in a salad dressing bottle. To get around, cholesterol hitchhikes on proteins. These combinations of fats and proteins are called lipoproteins. There are two main types you need to care about, and they have very different jobs. If you have ever looked at a blood test result, you have seen these acronyms: **HDL** and **LDL**. Let's break down exactly what they are doing while you go about your day.

First, let's talk about **Low-Density Lipoprotein**, or **LDL**. In the health world of the 1990s, we call this the "Bad" cholesterol. Think of LDL as the delivery truck. Its job is to carry cholesterol from the liver out to the cells that need it for repairs and hormone production. This sounds like a good thing, and it is—up to a point. The issue is that LDL is a bit of a messy delivery driver. If there is too much of it circulating in your system, it starts to drop its cargo along the walls of your arteries. It's like a truck with a leaky tailgate. Over time, that spilled cholesterol reacts with oxygen and other substances to form a thick, hard substance called **plaque**. This process is known as atherosclerosis. As that plaque builds up, the interior of the artery becomes narrower and narrower. It's exactly like a pipe in an old house getting filled with mineral deposits. Eventually, the opening becomes so small that a clot could get stuck, or the flow of blood becomes a mere trickle. This is how heart attacks and strokes begin.

On the other side of the field, we have **High-Density Lipoprotein**, or **HDL**. This is the “Good” cholesterol, and you want as much of this as you can get. If LDL is the messy delivery truck, HDL is the street sweeper. It cruises through your bloodstream, picks up the excess cholesterol that the LDL dropped, and carries it back to the liver to be broken down and removed from the body. A high level of HDL is like having a top-tier maintenance crew working twenty-four hours a day to keep your arterial superhighways clear and smooth. This is why when you get your blood work back, your doctor isn’t just looking at the total number. They are looking at the ratio. You want low LDL to prevent the mess and high HDL to clean up whatever spills happen. It’s a delicate balance that determines how healthy your cardiovascular system will be ten, twenty, or thirty years from now.

### The Danger of the Narrow Path

Why does this narrowing matter so much? It comes down to physics. When an artery narrows due to plaque buildup, the blood has to move faster and with more force to get through the gap. This raises your blood pressure. Furthermore, those plaques are not always stable. Sometimes, a piece of plaque can rupture, creating a rough surface that triggers your body’s clotting mechanism. A blood clot forms instantly to “heal” the rupture, but because the artery is already narrow, the clot can completely block the flow of blood. If this happens in a vessel supplying the heart, it’s a heart attack. If it happens in a vessel going to the brain, it's a stroke. This is why managing your cholesterol levels is about more than just numbers on a page; it is about keeping the path clear so your body can function without the constant threat of a structural failure.

Many people assume that they would feel it if their arteries were clogging, but that is a dangerous myth. You can have significant plaque buildup and feel completely fine—until you don't. High cholesterol is often called a silent condition because it doesn't cause a headache or a rash. The only way to know what is happening is to get tested and then take proactive steps to influence those numbers through your daily habits. Fortunately, we have some incredible tools in our nutritional arsenal that can help you manipulate these levels in your favor.

## The 90s Wellness Strategy: The Fiber First Protocol

Now that you know the players, how do we actually change the score? In the current landscape of health and nutrition, one of our most powerful weapons against high cholesterol is not a fancy pill or a complicated medical procedure. It is something you can find in the grocery store for a few cents a serving: **soluble fiber**. While we have known for a long time that fiber is good for digestion, we are now realizing that it plays a massive role in cleaning up your blood. This is the foundation of what I call the "Fiber First" Protocol.

There are two types of fiber: insoluble and soluble. Insoluble fiber is the "roughage" found in wheat bran and vegetable skins that keeps your digestive tract moving. But soluble fiber, found in foods like oats, beans, barley, and some fruits, is the real hero for your heart. When you eat soluble fiber, it turns into a gel-like substance in your intestines. This gel acts like a giant sponge, soaking up cholesterol and bile acids (which are made of cholesterol) before they can be reabsorbed into your bloodstream. Instead of that cholesterol going back into circulation to cause trouble, it gets trapped in the fiber and escorted right out of your body as waste. It is a natural "mop-up" operation that happens every time you sit down to a high-fiber meal.

One of the best sources of this "magic" fiber is the humble oat. If you start your day with a bowl of oatmeal, you are essentially sending a cleaning crew into your digestive system before you even head out the door. Studies have shown that just five to ten grams of soluble fiber and a piece of fruit. By making this a daily habit, you are consistently lowering the amount of raw material available for plaque formation. It is a simple, low-cost, and highly effective way to protect your longevity.

### HDL-Boosting Activity

While fiber is great at lowering the "Bad" LDL, we also need to focus on raising the "Good" HDL. Diet plays a role here, but the absolute best way to boost your HDL levels is through **regular aerobic exercise**. When you get your heart rate up into that target zone we discussed in earlier chapters, your body actually increases the production of those helpful HDL particles. Think of exercise as the fuel that keeps your "street sweepers" running. A sedentary lifestyle allows the HDL levels to sag, which means even a small amount of LDL can become a big problem because there is no one there to clean it up. By combining a high-fiber diet with consistent physical activity, you are attacking the problem from both ends: lowering the gunk and increasing the cleanup crew.

This dual approach is the gold standard for heart health in the 1990s. We aren't just trying to avoid "fatty" foods; we are actively adding "functional" foods and behaviors that change the chemistry of our blood. It is a proactive mindset. Instead of living in fear of your next blood test, you are taking specific, measurable actions every day to ensure that your arteries stay as clear as a mountain stream. It is about being the boss of your own biology.

## The Heart Through Time: The 1950s Seven Countries Study

Seven Countries Study, one of the most influential pieces of nutritional research in history.

Keys and his team followed the diets and health outcomes of thousands of men in seven different nations: the United States, Finland was a direct, undeniable link between the amount of saturated fat a population ate and their rate of heart disease. In places like Japan and the Mediterranean (specifically Greece and Italy), where the diet was low in animal fats and high in vegetables, grains, and unsaturated oils, heart disease was rare. In places like Finland and the United States, where butter, lard, and fatty meats were staples, the rates of heart attacks were through the roof.

This study was the "smoking gun" that pointed the finger at saturated fat as the primary driver of high cholesterol. It led to the realization that the western diet, which we once thought was a sign of prosperity and health, was actually clogging our collective arteries. This discovery sparked the low-fat revolution that we are still in the middle of today. It gave us the evidence we needed to say that what 1950s—we now know that things like sugar and stress also play huge roles—the fundamental lesson of the Seven Countries Study remains: the fats you choose matter.

### The Shift in Global Perception

Before the mid-20th century, a "rich" diet full of cream and meat was a status symbol. If you could afford to eat like a king, you did. But the Seven Countries Study showed that "eating like a king" was a East Asia. We began to see that the real "luxury" was a long, healthy life, and that meant trading in the heavy saturated fats for the life-extending power of plants, grains, and lean proteins. This historical shift is what paved the way for the advice I am giving you now. We are standing on the shoulders of decades of research that all points in one direction: clear arteries require a conscious choice about the fats we consume.

It is also who adopted the eating patterns of the lower-risk countries saw their own risks drop. This was a message of hope. It meant that even if your father and grandfather had heart trouble, you could write a different story for yourself by changing your relationship with the "C" word. You have the power to influence your internal environment through the choices you make at every single meal.

### Common Mistakes: The 'No Cholesterol' Trap

As we have become more aware of our health, the food industry has responded by plastering labels on everything they sell. But you have to be a savvy consumer, because some of these labels are designed to mislead you. One of the biggest mistakes people make is thinking that a label saying **"No Cholesterol"** automatically means the food is healthy for your heart. This is a classic 90s marketing trick, and I want you to be smarter than the advertisers.

Cholesterol is only found in animal products. Therefore, things like vegetable oil, potato chips, and sugary candies are naturally cholesterol-free. But just because a bag of chips has "No Cholesterol" on the front doesn't mean it isn't hurting your heart. Those chips are often fried in oils that are high in **saturated fats** or **trans fats**. Your liver takes those fats and uses them to manufacture LDL cholesterol. So, even though you aren't "eating" cholesterol directly from the chip, you are eating the raw materials that cause your body to overproduce the "Bad" kind. Always look past the big, bold claims on the front and check the nutrition facts panel on the back for the saturated fat content. That is where the real story is told.

People try to live on a diet of plain pasta and fat-free snacks. This is a mistake for two reasons. First, as we discussed, you need some fat for your brain and hormones to function. Second, many "fat-free" foods are type of fat in the blood that can contribute to artery clogging. The goal isn't "zero fat"; it's "smart fat." You want to replace the "Bad" saturated fats (found in butter, red meat, and full actually help lower your LDL and protect your heart.

## Ignoring the Role of Genetics

Finally, we have to address the "Genetics Trap." Sometimes, a person can do everything right—eat the oatmeal, run the miles, avoid the steak—and still have high cholesterol. This is because your body's internal "thermostat" for cholesterol production is partly determined by your DNA. Some people have a condition called familial hypercholesterolemia, where their liver simply produces too much cholesterol regardless and isn't working hard enough; it is just how your body is wired.

However, having a genetic predisposition makes your lifestyle choices **more** important, not less. If your body is already inclined to make too much LDL, you cannot afford to add more to the fire by eating a high-saturated-fat diet. You have to be even more diligent about your fiber intake and your exercise routine to help your system manage the load. Think of it like on top of oil changes. You can still drive that car for a long time, but you have to be a more attentive owner. Never use your genes as an excuse to give up on your heart-healthy habits.

### Your Action Plan: Clearing the Path

It is time to move from theory to practice. You don't need to overhaul your entire life overnight. In fact, small, consistent changes are much more likely to stick and produce long-term results. Here are three specific, actionable steps you can take today to start clearing those arterial superhighways and boosting your "Good" cholesterol levels.

1. **Swap your morning bagel for a bowl of oatmeal.** This is the easiest way to put the "Fiber First" Protocol into action. A standard bagel is mostly refined white flour, which does very little for your heart. By switching to oatmeal, you are getting a massive dose of soluble fiber right at the start of your day. If you find plain oatmeal boring, don't reach for the sugar bowl. Add a handful of blueberries or a sliced banana for extra fiber and flavor, or. It's like giving your arteries a gentle scrubbing every morning.

2. **Read one food label and find the 'Saturated Fat' line.** Knowledge is power. The next time you are in the kitchen or the grocery store, pick up a package of something you eat regularly—maybe it's your favorite crackers, a tub of margarine, or a frozen dinner. Ignore the marketing on the front. Flip it over and look at the "Saturated Fat" line on the nutrition label. If a serving has more than 2 or 3 grams of saturated fat, it's probably something you should eat only occasionally. Look for an alternative that is lower in saturated fat. This simple habit of "auditing" your food will make you much more aware of the hidden heart-cloggers in your diet.

3. Eat one serving of legumes today with protein, low in fat, and, most importantly, they are loaded with soluble fiber. One half-cup of black beans or lentils provides about the same amount of soluble fiber as a bowl of oatmeal. You can toss some chickpeas into a salad, add lentils to a soup, or have a side of black beans with your dinner. By making legumes a regular part of your rotation, you are providing your body with the tools it needs to mop up excess cholesterol throughout the day.

### Monitoring Your Progress

As you implement these steps, I want you to think about your current "Good" to "Bad" cholesterol ratio. If you haven't had a blood test recently, make an appointment to get one. You need a baseline so you can see how much progress you are making. When you get the results, don't just look at the "Total Cholesterol" number. Look at the HDL and LDL specifically. Are you eating enough fiber to clear your system? Are you moving your body enough to keep those "street sweepers" active? These are the questions that will guide your journey toward longevity.

Remember, your body is incredibly resilient. Even if you have spent years eating a diet high in saturated fats and ignoring your fiber intake, it is never too late to start clearing the path. The moment you start making better choices, your body begins to respond. Your liver starts to recalibrate, your HDL starts to climb, and the process of plaque buildup can slow down or even stabilize. You are not a passenger in this process; you are the driver. By understanding the chemistry of your blood and the power of your plate, you are taking the most important step any human can take: you are choosing to live a longer, more vibrant life.

In the coming weeks, pay attention to how you feel as you make these swaps. Many people find that as they clear the "gunk" out of their system, they have more energy and feel lighter. This isn't just in your head; it's because your heart is able to do its job more efficiently. Every beat is moving blood through clear, flexible pipes instead of pushing it through a clogged-up system. That is the feeling of a heart that is being cared for. That is the feeling of a path that has been cleared for the long haul. Keep focusing on that fiber, keep an eye on those fats, and keep moving. Your future self will thank you for the work you are doing right now.

Take a look at your next meal. Is there a way to add a little more fiber? Can you swap out a saturated fat for a heart-healthy one? These small decisions, made day after day, are what build a legacy of health. You have the information, you have the strategy, and you have the motivation. Now, go out there and show your heart some respect. Let's make sure those arterial superhighways stay open for business for a long, long time.

# Chapter 8
## The Low-Fat Frontier: 90s Nutritional Wisdom

Let's talk about the fuel you put into your machine. If you want to reach the finish line of a long, healthy life, you have to be honest about what is on the end of your fork. In the current world of health, there is one word that sends a shiver down the spine of every plates, and for good reason. For years, the average American diet has been swimming in oils, lards, and heavy creams - fat frontier, and it is simpler than you might expect. It is all about numbers, choices, and a little bit of common sense.

When we look at the basic building blocks of nutrition—protein, carbohydrates, and fat—one of these things is not like the others. While protein and carbs each pack about four calories into every gram, fat is a different beast entirely. It carries a whopping nine calories per gram. That is more than double the energy density of the other two. Imagine you are trying to pack a suitcase for a long trip. If you fill it with lead weights instead of cotton shirts, that the only thing it can: it stores it for later.

Now, I am not suggesting that fat is some kind of poison. Your body actually uses it for some pretty important jobs, like absorbing vitamins and protecting your nerves. But in our modern world, we aren't suffering from a lack of fat; we are drowning in it. Most of us are carrying around a heavy biological tax that our hearts have to pay every single second of every single day. If you want to lighten that load and give your ticker a fighting chance, you have to become a master of the low-fat lifestyle. This isn't about deprivation or eating cardboard; it is about being smarter than the average consumer and making substitutions that add up to massive gains in longevity over the long haul.

### Anatomy 101: The Hidden Weight on Your Heart

To understand why fat is such a big deal, we have to look under the hood. Most people think of fat as just the stuff they can pinch around their waistline or under their arms. That is what we call subcutaneous fat. While it might bother you when you look in the mirror or try to squeeze into your favorite pair of jeans, it isn't the most dangerous player itself around your internal organs like a heavy, suffocating blanket. It crowds your liver, your kidneys, and most importantly, it puts a massive amount of pressure on your cardiac muscle.

When you have an excess of visceral fat, your heart has to work against a physical barrier. Every time it beats, it is pushing against that internal pressure. But the problem goes even deeper than just physical space. Fat tissue is not just an inert storage tank; it is metabolically active. It releases chemicals into your bloodstream that can increase inflammation and make your blood vessels less flexible. Imagine trying to pump water through a hose fat. It has to generate more force just to move the same amount of blood, which leads to a thicker, less efficient heart muscle over time.

This internal crowding also affects your lungs. When your abdominal cavity is full of visceral fat, your diaphragm cannot drop down as far as it should when you take a deep breath. This means you aren't getting as much oxygen into your system with every inhale. Since your heart and lungs work as a team, a struggle for the lungs becomes a struggle for the heart. Your pulse has to quicken just to compensate for the lower oxygen levels. By reducing the amount of fat in your diet and burning off that internal storage, you are quite literally giving your organs room to breathe. You are removing the weights from the scale and letting your body function the way nature intended.

### The Problem with Density

Let's go back to those nine calories per gram for a second. The reason this matters so much for your heart health is that it makes it incredibly easy to overeat without even realizing it. You could eat a massive pile of steamed broccoli or a giant bowl of air-popped popcorn and only consume a hundred calories. But if you take a single tablespoon of butter or oil, you are already at that same hundred-calorie mark. Because fat is so small for how much energy it carries, it doesn't trigger the "fullness" sensors in your stomach the same way bulkier foods do. You can energy for the entire day.

When that excess energy enters your system, your liver has to process it. If it can't be used immediately for exercise or basic bodily functions, it gets packaged into triglycerides and sent out into the bloodstream. This makes your blood "thicker" and stickier in the short term, and in the long term, it leads to those fat deposits around your organs that we just talked about. This is why fat gram counting became such a vital tool in the 90s. If you can keep your fat intake to less than thirty percent of your total calories—and ideally even lower—you are cutting off the supply line for visceral fat. You are making it much harder for your body to store that internal "clutter" that gets in the way of your heart's performance.

**The 90s Wellness Strategy: The Substitution Game**

So, how do we actually do this without losing our minds? In the 90s, we have perfected a method called the Substitution Game. This isn't about going on a "diet" that lasts for two weeks and then failing. This is about a permanent shift in how you navigate the grocery store and your own kitchen. The goal is to find the high-fat items you love and swap them for lower-fat alternatives that give you the same satisfaction without the cardiac cost. It is a game of inches, and if you play it right, you can save thousands of fat grams every year.

The first and easiest place to start is the dairy aisle. For decades, we were told that whole milk was the gold standard. But a single glass of whole milk contains about eight grams of fat, and five of those are saturated—the kind that clogs your pipes. If you switch to two-percent milk, you cut that fat in half. If you go to one-percent, you cut it again. And if you make the jump to skim milk, you are getting all the calcium and protein with virtually zero fat. At first, skim milk might taste a little thin if you are used to the heavy stuff, but your taste buds will adjust within a week. Suddenly, whole milk will taste like heavy cream to you. This one swap alone can save you pounds of fat over the course of a year if you are a regular milk drinker.

Another classic move in the Substitution Game involves your favorite toppings. Do you love a baked potato with a big dollop of sour cream? Most people do. But sour cream is essentially pure milk fat. Try swapping it for non-fat plain yogurt. If you add a little bit of chopped chives or a dash of black pepper, the texture and tang are almost identical, but you've just eliminated almost all the fat from that meal. The same goes for mayonnaise on your sandwiches. Switch to a fat-free version or, better yet, use spicy mustard. Mustard has zero fat and adds a huge punch of flavor that mayo just can't match. These aren't sacrifices; they are upgrades for your arteries.

### Mastering the Art of Flavor Without Oil

One of the biggest hurdles people face on the low-fat frontier is the belief that fat equals flavor. We've been conditioned to think that if a food isn't glistening with oil or butter, it's going to be bland. I am here to tell you that is a myth. Flavor comes from spices, herbs, acids like lemon juice and vinegar, and the natural sugars in vegetables. Fat just coats your tongue and actually dulls your ability to taste the subtle notes in your food. When you start "Steaming for Flavor," you unlock a whole new world of culinary experiences.

Steaming is one of the most underutilized tools in the heart-healthy kitchen. When you fry a piece of fish or a chicken breast in a pan with oil, you are adding hundreds of unnecessary calories. But when you steam that same protein with a few slices of ginger, some garlic, and a splash of soy sauce, the meat stays moist and picks up all those aromatics without a single drop of grease. You can do the same with vegetables. Instead of sautéing your carrots in butter, steam them until they are tender-crisp and then hit them with a squeeze of fresh orange juice and a sprinkle of dill. The brightness of the citrus will wake up your palate in a way that butter never could.

## The Heart Through Time:

## The Rise of the Food Guide Pyramid

To nutritional advice has evolved. For a long time, the government used a simple "Basic Four" food groups model that gave equal weight to meat and dairy as it did to fruits and vegetables. But as heart disease rates continued to climb throughout the middle of the century. This led to the creation of the USDA Food Guide Pyramid, which was released to the public in 1992.

The Pyramid was a revolutionary shift in thinking. For the first time, we had a visual representation that put grains, breads, and cereals at the very bottom—the widest part of the structure. This was the foundation. The message was clear: your sections for meat and dairy. And way up at the very tip, in the smallest triangle possible, were the fats, oils, and sweets. The Pyramid told the American public that fat should be a tiny "extra" in our lives, not a main attraction.

This shift was based on the understanding that the most heart-healthy societies in the world—like those in the Mediterranean or rural Asia—rely on a grain-based diet. When you build your meals around rice, pasta, or whole-wheat bread, you are filling up on fiber and complex energy that burns slowly and cleanly. You aren't loading your blood with the heavy triglycerides that come from a meat-heavy, fat-heavy diet. The 90s focus on the "grain base" isn't just a trend; it is a return to a more natural way of eating that supports the heart's long-term health. It emphasizes volume and energy without the dense caloric baggage of fat.

### The Lesson of the Mediterranean

While the Pyramid gave us a great structure, we also looked at specific cultures that seemed to have the secret to longevity. Researchers in the 90s have spent a lot of time studying people in places like Crete and southern Italy. What they found was that these people ate very little red meat and almost no butter. Their fat came primarily from plant sources like olive oil, and even then, it was used sparingly compared to the way we use fats in the West. Their plates were dominated by beans, lentils, crusty breads, and an abundance of fresh produce.

The result? These populations had some of the lowest rates of heart disease in the world, despite not having access to high-tech gyms or advanced cardiac medications. Their "medicine" was their diet. They were naturally playing the Substitution Game before it even had a name. By following the logic of the Food Guide Pyramid and focusing on that wide base of plant-based foods, we are trying to replicate those results in our own lives. We are learning that you, the more energy you often have to tackle your day and your workouts.

### Common Mistakes: The 'Fat-Free' Cookie Trap

Now, I have to give you a warning. Whenever a new health trend takes over, the food industry finds a way to exploit it, and the low-fat movement is no exception. We are currently seeing a flood of products on grocery store shelves labeled "Fat-Free." You see fat-free cookies, fat-free cakes, and fat-free crackers. It sounds like a dream come true, right? You can eat all the treats you want and your heart will be fine? Not so fast. This is one of the biggest mistakes people make on the low-fat frontier.

Here is the secret: when food companies take the fat out of a cookie, they have to put something else in to make it taste good and keep its texture. Usually, that "something else" is a massive amount of sugar. While sugar doesn't have the same calorie density as fat, eating liver can actually convert excess sugar into the very triglycerides we are trying to avoid. If you sit down and eat an entire box of fat You are still putting a strain on your system. A "fat-free" label is not a green light to overindulge; it is just a tool to help you make better choices in moderation.

Another common error is trying to eliminate every single molecule of fat from your life. As I mentioned earlier, your body does need some essential fatty acids to function. Things like Omega-3 and Omega-6 fats, found in fish and certain nuts, are actually good for your heart because they help reduce inflammation. If you go on a "zero-fat" diet, your skin will get dry, your hair will get brittle, and you might even find it harder to concentrate. The goal is to eliminate the "garbage" fats—the saturated fats in burgers and the trans fats in processed snack cakes—while keeping a small amount of the "smart" fats. Don't throw the baby out with the bathwater. Just be very selective about which fats get an invite to the party.

### The Danger of Thinking All Fats are the Same

In our rush to be heart-healthy, it is easy to lump all fats into one "bad" category. But that actually improve your cholesterol profile. The fat in the pizza is saturated and often comes with a side of sodium that sends your blood pressure through the roof.

When you are looking at a food label, don't just look at the "Total Fat" line. Look at the breakdown. If most of that fat is coming from "Saturated Fat" or "Trans Fat," put it back on the shelf. If it is mostly "Monounsaturated" or "Polyunsaturated," and the total amount is reasonable, then it can have a place in your diet. This nuance is what separates the beginners from the experts. An loaded with thirty grams of sugar is a cardiac disaster waiting to happen. Use your head, read the labels, and don't be fooled by flashy marketing.

### Your Action Plan: Conquering the Frontier

It is time to take these principles and put them into practice in your own kitchen. You don't need a culinary degree to be a heart-healthy cook; you just need the right tools and a plan. Here are three specific steps you can take this week to start reducing the fat load on your heart and mastering the Substitution Game.

1. **Buy a high-quality non-stick pan.** If you only take one thing away from this chapter, let it be this: your cookware matters. A good non-stick surface allows you to cook eggs, chicken, and vegetables with little to no oil. If you are using an old, scratched-up stainless steel pan, you are probably dumping a tablespoon of oil in every time you cook just to keep the food from sticking. That is an extra hundred calories you don't need. By investing in a solid non-stick pan, you are giving yourself the ability to sear and sauté without the fat. It is the single best investment you can make for your kitchen and your heart.

2. **Replace one 'fried' meal this week with a 'broiled' or 'steamed' version.** We all have our favorite comfort foods. Maybe it's fried chicken on Sundays or fried fish on Fridays. I am asking you to pick just one of those meals this week and change the cooking method. Instead of breading and frying that chicken, try seasoning it with herbs and lemon and popping it under the broiler. You still get a great crust, but you aren't adding any grease. If you usually have fried potatoes, try steaming some small red potatoes and tossing them with fresh parsley and a tiny bit of olive oil. You will be surprised at how much cleaner you feel after a meal that hasn't been submerged in a fryer.

3. **Try a non-fat version of your favorite dairy product.** Whether it is milk, yogurt, or cottage cheese, make the switch to a non-fat or week after. Your taste buds are remarkably adaptable, and they will learn to appreciate the lighter, cleaner taste of low-fat dairy. Remember, every gram of fat you don't eat is a gram of fat your heart doesn't have to deal with.

### Monitoring Your Progress

As you start making these substitutions, pay attention to how your body responds. Many people find that within just a few weeks of cutting back on fat, their energy levels become much more stable. You won't have that "heavy" feeling after lunch that makes you want to take a nap. That is because your body isn't spending all its energy trying to process a massive load of lipids. You are running on clean-burning fuel, and your heart is loving every minute of it.

You might also notice that your clothes start to fit a little better. Remember, fat is the most calorie-dense nutrient. When you cut it out, your total calorie intake drops significantly, even if you are eating the same volume of food. This is the "secret" to sustainable weight loss and heart health. You don't have to eat less food; you just have to eat less fat. By filling your plate with the base of the Food Guide Pyramid—grains, fruits, and vegetables—you can stay full and satisfied while your body burns through its internal stores of visceral fat. You are reclaiming the space inside your own body.

### The Long-Term Vision

The low-fat frontier is not a place you visit for a week and then leave. It is a new way of living a vote for your future self. You are deciding that you want to be the person who can still go for a brisk walk or play with your grandkids twenty or thirty years from now. You are deciding that your heart is worth more than the fleeting taste of a greasy burger.

Think about the hidden fat that sneaks into your diet. Is it in the creamer you put in your coffee? Is it in the "healthy" salad dressing that is actually eighty percent oil? Once you start looking, you will see these opportunities for substitution everywhere. And each one is a victory. Don't get discouraged if you slip up and have a high-fat meal every now and then. The goal isn't perfection; it is consistency. If eighty percent of your choices are low-fat and heart-smart, you are already miles ahead of the average person.

We are living in an era of incredible discovery when it comes to nutrition. We have the data, we have the tools, and we have the motivation to change our destiny. Your heart has been working for you since before you were born, never taking a single second off. Doesn't it deserve a little bit of help? By mastering the low-fat frontier, you are giving your heart the greatest gift possible: a clear path and a lighter load. You are taking ownership of the engine that keeps you alive. So, let's keep playing the game, making the swaps, and building a body that is lean, mean, and ready for the long haul. Your heart is waiting for you to lead the way.

Take a look at your pantry right now. Are there "fat traps" lurking in there? Can you find a way to make your next dinner just a little bit lighter? These small, daily decisions are the bricks that build a fortress of health around your heart. You have the knowledge, you have the plan, and you have the drive. Now, go out there and conquer the low-fat frontier. Your heart is counting on you, and I know you can do it. Let's make every calorie count for something good.

# Chapter 9
## Sodium:
## The Silent Pressure Cooker

Imagine your circulatory system as a complex network of plumbing. In a perfect world, the water flows smoothly, the pipes stay clear, and the pressure remains at a steady, manageable level. But what happens if you suddenly double the amount of fluid trying to squeeze through those same pipes? The pressure spikes. The joints start to strain. The pump at the center of the system has to strain against the resistance, pounding away just to keep things moving. This is exactly what over the years, it turns your body into a high-pressure environment that can eventually lead to a blowout.

Most of us don't even think about salt until we realize we've forgotten it. We reach for that little glass shaker out of habit, dusting our eggs, our potatoes, and our steaks before we've even taken a single bite. We've been trained to believe that salt is the primary source of flavor, the essential ingredient that makes food worth eating. But in our modern world, salt has shifted from a rare mineral to a ubiquitous additive that is hiding in places you would never expect. It is in your cereal, your bread, your canned peas, and your "healthy" frozen dinners. This overabundance is creating a national health crisis, and it is time we pulled back the curtain on this mineral to see what it is really doing to our cardiovascular health.

The goal here isn't to make your heart the relief it deserves. By understanding the mechanics of how sodium interacts with your blood and your cells, you can make informed choices that prolong your life. We are talking about moving away from the "salt-heavy" habits of the past and embracing a fresh, vibrant way of eating that relies on the natural brightness of herbs and spices. It is a shift in perspective that will leave you feeling lighter, more energetic, and far more in control of your physical destiny.

### Anatomy 101: The Biology of the Squeeze

To really get why sodium is such a big deal, we have to talk about a process called osmosis. This is a fundamental law of biology that dictates how water moves in and out of your cells. In simple terms, water follows salt. Your body maintains a very specific balance of electrolytes in your bloodstream to keep everything functioning. When you consume a large amount of sodium, it enters your blood, and your body reacts by trying to dilute that salt to maintain the proper concentration. It does this by pulling water out of your cells and into your blood vessels.

This is where the trouble starts. When that extra water enters your bloodstream, your total blood volume increases. It is like trying to force two gallons of liquid into a one-gallon container. Your arteries and veins are flexible to a point, but they can only stretch so far. As the volume goes up, the force against the walls of your blood vessels increases. This is the literal definition of high blood pressure, or hypertension. Every time your heart beats, it has to push against this increased resistance. Over months and years, this constant "squeeze" causes the walls of your arteries to become thick and stiff. They>But the damage doesn't stop with the pressure. High sodium levels also put a massive burden on your kidneys. These organs act as the filtration system for your body, constantly working to remove excess minerals and waste products. When you are constantly flooding and less efficient. When your kidneys can't keep up, even more fluid stays in your system, and your blood pressure climbs even higher. It is a systemic issue that affects your entire body, but the heart is always the one that pays the ultimate price for this internal flood.

There is also the issue of "hidden" edema. Have you ever noticed that your rings feel tight or your ankles look a bit swollen after a particularly salty meal at a restaurant? That is your body holding onto water in its tissues. While the swelling in your feet might be an annoyance, the swelling in your vascular system is a silent threat. You can't feel your blood pressure rising the way you can feel a headache or a muscle cramp. That is why doctors call hypertension the "silent killer." You might feel perfectly fine while your heart is struggling to pump against a tide of salt-water. By the time symptoms actually appear, the damage to your arteries is often already significant.

## The Flavor Revolution: The Herb and Spice Overhaul

Now, let's get practical. If we want to lower the pressure, we have to lower the salt. But for most people, the idea of "low-sodium" food conjures up images of bland, unappealing meals. In the 90s, we are moving past that outdated way of thinking. We are entering the era of the **Herb and Spice Overhaul**. This is about learning to season your food with intention rather than just reaching for the shaker out of boredom. Your tongue has about ten thousand taste buds, and they are capable of detecting a massive range of flavors. Salt just happens to be the loudest one, so it tends to drown out everything else.

When you reduce your salt intake, something amazing happens: your taste buds actually become more sensitive. Within about two weeks of cutting back, you will start to notice the natural sweetness years with a layer of sodium. The **Herb and Spice Overhaul** is your way of rediscovering what food actually tastes like. It is a culinary awakening that makes your meals more interesting while protecting your arteries.

One of the best tools in your new flavor kit is acidity. Think about how a squeeze of fresh lemon juice wakes up a piece of grilled fish or a bowl of steamed vegetables. The acid provides a "brightness" that mimics the sharp hit of salt without any of the cardiovascular consequences. Vinegars are another secret weapon. Balsamic, red wine, and apple cider vinegars can add depth and complexity to soups, stews, and salads. If a dish feels like it is "missing something," don't reach for the salt. Reach for a lime, a lemon, or a bottle of high-quality vinegar. You will be shocked at how much better the food tastes when the natural flavors are allowed to shine.

Then, there are the aromatics. Garlic and onions are the foundation of great cooking around the world, and for good reason. They provide a savory "umami" punch that satisfies the palate in a way that salt alone never could. Whether you are roasting whole cloves of garlic until they are sweet and spreadable or sautéing onions until they are caramelized and golden, you are building flavor from the ground up. Combine these with fresh herbs like rosemary, thyme, basil, and cilantro, and you have an infinite palette of tastes to work with. These plants aren't just for garnish; they are powerful flavor agents that can transform a basic chicken breast into a gourmet meal.

If you like a bit of a kick, spices are your best friend. Black pepper, cumin, paprika, and chili powder add heat and interest to your meals. When your tongue is busy processing the tingle of a spicy pepper or the warmth of cinnamon, it doesn't miss the salt. Experimenting with different spice blends—like a salt-free curry powder or a Mediterranean herb mix—can keep your diet from feeling repetitive. This is the heart of the strategy: replacing a one-dimensional seasoning (salt) with a multi-dimensional world of flavor. It takes a little more effort than just shaking a glass jar, but your heart will thank you for it every single day.

## The Heart Through Time: From Currency to Chemical

It is interesting to consider how our relationship with salt has changed throughout human history. For thousands of years, salt was one of the most precious substances on Earth. In ancient times, it was so valuable that it was used as currency. In fact, the word "salary" comes from the Latin word *salarium*, which was the money given to Roman soldiers so they could buy salt. It was essential for survival because it was the only way to preserve meat and fish before the invention of refrigeration. Without salt, civilization as we know it might not have been able to expand across the globe.

Back then, humans had to work hard to get enough sodium. It was mined from the earth or evaporated from seawater in a labor-intensive process. Our bodies evolved to be incredibly efficient at holding onto salt because it was so scarce in the natural environment. We developed a biological "salt hunger" that drove us to seek out this mineral to maintain our electrolyte balance. In those days, a high-salt diet was almost impossible for the average person to achieve. Most of our ancestors were likely eating a diet that was naturally very low in sodium, consisting mostly of fresh plants and occasional game meats.

Fast forward to the modern era, and the situation has flipped completely. With the industrial revolution and the rise of mass-produced food, salt became incredibly cheap and easy to manufacture. Food companies discovered that salt is a miracle worker for processed goods. It acts as a preservative, extending shelf life for months or even years. It masks the bitter metallic tastes that can come from canning processes. And perhaps most importantly, it is addictive. The more salt people eat, the more they want, which keeps them coming back for more of those salty snacks and pre-packaged meals.

We are now living in a world where our ancient biology is mismatched with our modern environment. We still have that evolutionary drive to seek out salt, but we are now surrounded by an unlimited supply of it. We are essentially "short-circuiting" our own systems. We are consuming ten, fifteen, or even twenty times the amount of sodium our ancestors did, but our bodies are still trying to hold onto every single milligram. This is why the rise of processed foods in the twentieth century directly correlates with the explosion of heart disease and stroke. We took a precious ancient resource and turned it into a cheap, dangerous additive that is slowly tightening the pressure on our hearts.

### The Sodium Rinse: Cleaning Up Your Kitchen

A huge part of the problem is that we often don't even know we are eating salt. Only about ten percent of the sodium. The remaining eighty percent? It comes from processed and restaurant foods. This is the "hidden" salt that is doing the most damage. To get your blood pressure under control, you have to become a detective in your own kitchen and learn the **Sodium Rinse** technique.

Canned goods are one of the biggest offenders. Whether it is beans, corn, or peas, the liquid in that can is usually packed with sodium to keep the vegetables firm and preserve their color. But you don't have to eat it. The **Sodium Rinse** is a simple but effective habit: whenever you open a can of vegetables or beans, dump them into a colander and run cold water over them for all the convenience of the canned food with a fraction of the cardiac cost. It is a small change that yields massive results over time.

You also need to look at your "staple" foods. Bread is a surprising source of hidden sodium. Because we eat so much of it, the salt adds up quickly. A single slice of white or whole-wheat bread can have as much as 150 to 200 milligrams of sodium. If you have a sandwich with two slices of bread, some deli meat, and a slice of cheese, you could easily be hitting. Look for "low-sodium" or "no-salt-added" versions of your favorite breads and crackers. You might find that the brand you've been buying for years is the worst offender on the shelf.

Breakfast cereals are another trap. Even the ones that market themselves as "healthy" or "heart-smart" can be loaded with sodium to balance out the sweetness. It is a common trick in the food industry: use salt to make sugar taste sweeter and use sugar to make salt less harsh. It is a flavor profile designed to keep you eating, but it is a disaster for your blood oatmeal or cream of wheat and add your own flavor with fresh berries and cinnamon. This way, you are the one in control of what goes into your body, not a food scientist in a laboratory.

## Common Mistakes: The Sea Salt Myth

One of the most frequent errors I see people make is falling for the "natural" marketing of sea salt from exotic islands. The marketing suggests that because these salts contain "trace minerals," they are somehow healthier for your heart than standard table salt. I am here to tell you: that is a dangerous misconception. When it comes to your blood pressure, your body does not care where the sodium came from. Whether it was mined from an ancient cave or evaporated from the Pacific Ocean, sodium is sodium.

While sea salt might have a slightly different texture or a subtle mineral flavor, it still has the same chemical effect on your blood volume. If you use a teaspoon of sea salt, you are getting the same amount of sodium as a teaspoon of regular table salt. Don't let the fancy packaging fool you into thinking you can use it liberally. If you are trying to lower your pressure, you need to reduce your intake of *all* salts, regardless of their origin or color. The "trace minerals" in these salts are present in such tiny amounts that you would have to eat a lethal amount of salt to get any real nutritional benefit from them. Get your minerals from leafy greens and whole grains instead.

Another mistake is assuming that "low-sodium" means the same thing as "no-salt-added." These are legal terms with specific meanings. "Low-sodium" generally means the product has 140 milligrams or less per serving. This is a great choice. However, "Reduced Sodium" only means the product has twenty-five percent less salt than the original version. If the original version was a sodium bomb, the "reduced" version is still likely way too high for someone watching their heart health.

Always look at the actual numbers on the nutrition facts panel. Don't trust the big, flashy claims on the front of the box. The truth is always in the small print on the back.

Finally, watch out for the "sweet" trap. Many people think that if a food doesn't taste salty, it must be low in sodium. This is completely false. As I mentioned with bread and cereal, salt is often used as a background flavor enhancer in sweet foods. Chocolate bars, cookies, and even some sodas contain sodium to balance the flavor profiles. This is why it is so important to read labels on everything you buy, not just the savory snacks. You could be sabotaging your heart health before you even get to dinner just by eating "sweet" processed foods throughout the day.

### Your Action Plan: The Two-Week Reset

It is time to take the reins and start your journey toward a lower-pressure life. You don't have to change everything overnight, but you do need to start making conscious choices. Here are three specific, actionable steps you can take this week to begin the process of retraining your palate and protecting your arteries. These are the foundations of a heart-smart lifestyle.

1. **Remove the salt shaker from the dinner table.** This sounds simple, but it is incredibly powerful. Most of the salt we add to our food is added out of habit, not necessity. By moving the shaker to a high cupboard or into the pantry, you break the automatic "shake-shake" routine. If you find that you really need a flavor boost once you sit down to eat, try having a bowl of lemon wedges or a pepper grinder on the table instead. This one

change alone can significantly reduce your daily sodium intake without requiring you to change a single recipe.

2. **Rinse all canned beans and vegetables.** Make the **Sodium Rinse** a non-negotiable part of your kitchen routine. Keep a colander right next to your can opener. Whether you are making a salad, a soup, or a side dish, give those canned goods a good scrub under cold water. You will be washing away a massive amount of hidden sodium that would otherwise end up in your bloodstream. It takes ten extra seconds, but it provides a lifetime of benefits for your heart and kidneys.

3. **Check the sodium content of your favorite bread and cereal.** If your cereal is a sodium trap, you are creating a permanent downward shift in your blood pressure levels.

As you implement these steps, I want you to be patient with yourself. Your taste buds have been conditioned by years of high-salt eating. At first, things might taste a little "quiet." But I promise you, if you stick with it for just fourteen days, your palate will reset. You will start to find that processed foods taste unpleasantly salty, and you will begin to crave the fresh, clean flavors of whole foods. This is the moment you know you are winning. You are no longer a slave to the "salt hunger" of your ancestors; you are a modern, health-conscious individual who is in pressure cuff at home, start taking regular readings and keeping a log. You might be surprised at how quickly the numbers begin to drop once you cut out the excess sodium. Seeing that downward trend is the best motivation in the world. It is tangible proof that the work you are doing in the kitchen is having a direct, life-saving impact on your cardiovascular system. You aren't just eating better; you are literally restructuring the environment inside your blood vessels.

Think about the long-term vision for your life. Do you want to be the person who is limited by medication and later years? Your heart is a magnificent machine, but it isn't indestructible. It needs you to be its advocate. By turning down the "silent pressure cooker" of sodium, you are giving your heart the freedom to beat steadily and strongly for decades to come. You have the knowledge, you have the tools, and now you have the plan. Let's get to work and make every meal a victory for your heart.

Take a look in your pantry right now. Pick up one can or one box and look at that sodium number. Now you know exactly what it means and how to handle it. This is the beginning of a new chapter in your health journey. The road to a healthy heart is paved with fresh herbs, bright citrus, and a commitment to keeping the pressure under control. You are doing the best thing you can possibly do for your longevity. Keep going, stay focused, and enjoy the true flavors of a life well-lived.

# Chapter 10
## The Power of Produce: Vitamins for Vitality

Imagine for a second that you are standing in a lush, green field under the bright afternoon sun. All around you, the ground is bursting with life. From the deep red of a vine-ripened tomato to the sharp, electric green of a head of romaine lettuce, the earth is basically a giant, open-air pharmacy. It is a place where every leaf, stalk, and fruit is packed with specialized chemicals designed to keep a living system running at peak performance. For far too long, we have treated vegetables as the boring side dish that we have to choke down before we get to the "real" food. But if you want to keep your internal engine humming for the next several decades, it is time to start seeing these plants for what they actually are: the high-octane fuel that keeps your cardiovascular system from rusting out from the inside.

The truth is that your body is constantly under attack. No, it is not just from the stress of your job or the smog in the air, though those things certainly don't help. I am talking about a biological process that happens every time you take a breath. As your body uses oxygen to create energy, it produces byproducts called free radicals. These are unstable molecules that bounce around your bloodstream like tiny pinballs, smashing into the delicate lining of your arteries. If left unchecked, this process leads to something called oxidation. You have seen oxidation in the real world; it is exactly what happens when a piece of iron is left out in the rain and turns into a pile of reddish-brown rust. When this happens inside your blood vessels, it creates a rough surface where cholesterol and fat can easily snag and start building up. This is the start of the "clogged pipe" scenario that every health-conscious person wants to avoid.

This is where the power of produce comes into play. Fruits and vegetables are loaded with antioxidants—nature's own rust-proofing system. These incredible compounds search out those rogue free radicals and neutralize them before they can do any damage to your circulatory highway. By filling your plate with a variety of plant life, you are essentially sending a maintenance crew into your veins to smooth out the walls and keep everything flowing without a hitch. It is a simple, effective, and delicious way to ensure that your heart stays as strong as a marathon runner's well into your golden years. Let's break down exactly how these vitamins work and why they are the secret weapon in your wellness arsenal.

## Anatomy 101: The Shield and the Spark

To understand why a salad is more than just a bowl of fiber, we need to look at the three heavy hitters of the vitamin world: Vitamin A, Vitamin C, and Vitamin E. These are the primary antioxidants that your heart relies on for protection. They work together as a team, each covering a different part of the defensive line. Vitamin A, often found in the form of beta-carotene in bright orange vegetables like carrots and sweet potatoes, is fantastic for maintaining the integrity of your cellular membranes. It acts as a primary barrier, making sure the cells that line your blood vessels stay tough and resilient against the constant pressure of your pulse.

Then we have Vitamin C. Most people. Vitamin C is water-soluble, meaning it travels through the fluid parts of your blood, catching free radicals in the "open water." It is also a key player in the production of collagen. While you might associate collagen with youthful skin, it is actually the "glue" that keeps your arteries flexible. As we age, our arteries can become stiff and brittle, which forces the heart to push harder to move blood through the system. A steady supply of Vitamin C ensures that those vessels remain elastic and supple, allowing them to expand and contract with every beat without cracking or scarring.

Rounding out the trio is Vitamin E. Unlike Vitamin C, this one is fat-soluble. It embeds itself directly into the fatty parts of your cell walls and the cholesterol particles floating in your blood. This is crucial because it prevents LDL cholesterol—the "bad" kind—from becoming oxidized. Plain form the plaques that lead to blockages. Vitamin E acts as a protective coating, keeping those fat particles from turning into a dangerous sludge. When you eat these three vitamins together, you are creating a multi-layered shield that protects every inch of your cardiovascular landscape.

But the benefits of produce go beyond just the letter-named vitamins. We also have to talk about two minerals that are the unsung heroes of your heart's electrical system: potassium and magnesium. Your heart is an electric pump, and it requires a very specific balance of minerals to fire its signals correctly. Potassium is the direct counter-balance to sodium. While sodium causes your body to hold onto water and raises your blood pressure, potassium encourages your kidneys to release excess fluid and helps your blood vessel walls relax. Magnesium, meanwhile, acts as a natural calcium channel blocker, helping the heart muscle to relax after every contraction. Without enough of these minerals, your heart can become irritable, leading to palpitations or a steady climb in your resting blood pressure. Luckily, the produce aisle is overflowing with both.

### The Five-a-Day Challenge

Now that you know the science, it is time to talk about the strategy. Back in the early 90s, the National Cancer Institute and various health organizations launched a massive campaign called "Five-a-Day for Better Health." The goal was simple: get every person to eat at least five servings of fruits and vegetables every single day. While the message was straightforward, the impact on heart health was revolutionary. By hitting this target, you aren't just getting your vitamins; you are also crowding out the processed, high-fat foods that often dominate the American dinner table. It is a game of nutritional displacement. If half your plate is covered in broccoli and peppers, there simply isn't as much room for the greasy fries or the heavy cream sauces.

I know what you are thinking. Five servings sounds like a lot of work. But a "serving" isn't as big as you might imagine. We aren't talking about five giant bowls of salad. A serving is generally about half a cup of chopped vegetables, one medium, the mountain becomes a molehill. It is about integrating these foods into the things you are already eating. It is about the "Antioxidant Loading" technique—finding every possible opportunity to sneak a plant into your meal. If you are having cereal in the morning, toss in a handful of blueberries. If you are making a sandwich for lunch, pile on the spinach and tomato until it is hard to close. These small additions add up to a massive cumulative benefit for your arteries.

One of the most effective ways to manage this is with the Color-Plate Method. This is a visual check that you are looking at a heart-health desert. You want to see a rainbow. The different colors in plants actually represent different types of protective phytonutrients. Red fruits like raspberries and strawberries are packed with anthocyanins that protect against inflammation. Yellow and orange produce, like squash and apricots, are rich in those carotenoids we talked about earlier. Deep greens are your source for lutein and folate. By aiming for a colorful plate, you are automatically ensuring a wide spectrum of nutritional protection without ever having to look at a complicated chart or a textbook.

To keep yourself on track, I highly recommend using a “Five-a-Day Tracker.” This can be a simple notepad on your refrigerator or a small card you keep in your wallet. Every time you eat a serving of produce, give yourself a checkmark. There is something incredibly satisfying about seeing those five marks lined up by the end of the day. It turns your nutrition into a winnable game. And don’t worry about being perfect from day one. If you are currently only eating one vegetable a day (and no, french fries don’t count!), aim for two tomorrow. Build your momentum slowly but surely. Your heart doesn’t need a sudden, unsustainable overhaul; it needs a steady, consistent supply of the good stuff to keep the rust away.

### The Heart Through History: The Mystery of the Sea

We can learn a lot about the power of vitamins by looking back at one of the most terrifying medical mysteries of the past.

For hundreds of years, the greatest threat to a sailor wasn't a storm or an enemy ship; it was a horrifying disease called scurvy. Men would set out on long voyages across the ocean, and within a few months, their bodies would literally start to fall apart. Their gums would bleed, their old wounds would reopen, and they would become so weak that their hearts would eventually give out. At the time, no one knew why this was happening. People thought it was caused by "bad air," "laziness," or even the wood of the ships themselves.

It wasn't until the mid-1700s that a Scottish naval surgeon named James Lind conducted what is often considered one of the first clinical trials in history. He took twelve sailors suffering from scurvy and divided them into pairs, giving each pair a different supplement. Some got cider, some got vinegar, and some got seawater. But the two lucky sailors who were given two oranges and a lemon every day made a miraculous recovery within just one week. They went from being nearly dead to being back on duty, while the others remained sick. Lind had discovered that there was something vital in fresh fruit that the human body absolutely required to stay alive.

Eventually, the British Royal Navy caught on and began issuing a daily ration of lime juice to every sailor, which earned them the nickname "limeys." We now know that the "magic" ingredient was Vitamin C. Because humans are one of the few animals on Earth that cannot produce our own Vitamin C, we are entirely dependent on getting it from our food. The sailors' hearts were failing because, without Vitamin C, their bodies couldn't produce the collagen necessary to keep their blood vessels and heart tissue together. Their circulatory systems were quite literally disintegrating from the inside out.

While we don't see full-blown scurvy very often in the modern world, many of us are living in a state of "subclinical" deficiency. We are getting just enough Vitamin C to keep our teeth from falling out, but not enough to keep our arteries in prime condition. We are like those sailors on a long voyage, slowly depleting our reserves while our cardiovascular systems struggle to maintain their structural integrity. By looking at the lessons of history, we can see that produce isn't just a "healthy choice"—it is a biological necessity. Those citrus fruits saved the lives of thousands of sailors, and the same vitamins can save yours by providing the raw materials your heart needs to stay strong and flexible for a lifetime.

### Common Mistakes to Avoid

When you start increasing your produce intake, it is easy to fall into a few common traps that can rob you of the benefits you are working so hard to achieve. The first is the "Boiling Blunder." We have all been to a dinner where the vegetables are cooked until they are a mushy, grey-green mess. While it might make them easier to chew, boiling vegetables in a large pot of water for a long time causes many of the vitamins—especially Vitamin C and the B vitamins—to leach out into the water. When you pour that water down the drain, you are literally throwing the heart-healthy part of the meal into the sewer. To keep those vitamins where they belong, try steaming, roasting, or quick-sautéing your vegetables. You want them to stay bright and have a little bit of a "snap" when you bite into them. This preserves the nutrients and the flavor.

Another big mistake is the "Juice Trap." A lot of people think that drinking a giant glass of orange or apple juice is the same as eating the fruit itself. While juice does have some vitamins, it is missing the most important part: the fiber. Fiber is what slows down the absorption of sugar into your bloodstream, preventing a spike in insulin that can actually be hard on your heart over time. Furthermore, the process of juicing often removes the peel and the pulp, which is where many of the most powerful antioxidants are stored. A glass of juice is essentially a dose of liquid sugar with a few vitamins sprinkled in. Whenever possible, choose the whole fruit. It is more filling, better for your digestion, and far more beneficial for your cholesterol levels.

Finally, don't let the "Fresh or Nothing" mentality it isn't worth eating. This simply isn't true. In many cases, frozen vegetables are actually more nutritious than the "fresh" ones that have been sitting in a shipping container for two weeks and then sitting on a grocery store shelf for another three days. Frozen produce is usually picked at the peak of ripeness and flash-frozen immediately, which locks in the vitamins of frozen bags in your freezer. They are a fantastic, heart-smart backup that ensures you never have an excuse to skip your permanent part of your life, you need to have a few "go-to" techniques in your kitchen. One of my favorites is "Antioxidant Loading." This is the practice of adding extra vegetables to every single dish you cook, even if they aren't in the original recipe. Making a meatloaf? Grate some carrots and zucchini into the mix. Making a pot of chili? Throw in some extra bell peppers and onions. The flavors will blend together beautifully, and you will be boosting the nutrient density of your meal without even noticing. It is a painless way to hit your daily goals while making your food taste richer and more complex.

Another powerful technique is "The Sunday Prep." One of the biggest barriers to eating produce is the time it takes to wash, peel, and chop. On a busy Tuesday evening, the last thing you want to do is spend twenty minutes prepping a head of broccoli. Instead, take an hour on Sunday afternoon to process your vegetables for the week. Wash your greens, chop your peppers, and peel your carrots. Store them in clear containers at eye-level in your refrigerator. When you open the fridge looking for a snack or getting ready to cook dinner, the healthy choices are right there, ready to go. Convenience is the key to consistency. If the healthy choice is also the easy choice, you are much more likely to stick with it.

Lastly, try the "New Veggie of the Week" approach. It is easy to get stuck in a rut of eating the same three vegetables over and over again. But remember, diversity is the key to getting a full range of antioxidants. you were a kid. Maybe it is a purple head of cauliflower, a bunch of Swiss chard, or a jicama. Look up a quick way to prepare it and give it a shot. You might discover a new favorite, and you will definitely be giving your heart a broader range of vitamin protection. Keeping your palate excited is one of the best ways to keep your healthy habits alive for the long haul.

### Your Action Plan: The Vitality Kickstart

It is time to move from theory to action. You have the knowledge, and you understand the high stakes for your cardiovascular health. Now, let's put these ideas into practice starting right now. You don't need a fancy diet plan or a personal chef to start protecting your arteries from "rust." You just need a commitment to the plants that the earth has provided for you. Here are three specific steps you can take this week to begin your journey toward a heart full of vitality.

1. **Eat one fruit or vegetable with every single meal today.** This is the simplest way to start your Five-a-Day journey. Don't worry about the total count just yet; just focus on the frequency. If you are having eggs for breakfast, have a piece of melon on the side. If you are having a turkey sandwich for lunch, add a side of baby carrots. For dinner, make sure there is a green vegetable on your plate. By making produce a non-negotiable part of every meal, you are establishing a new baseline for your health that will soon become second nature.

2. **Try a new "color" of produce this week.** Take a look at what you usually buy and identify a color that is missing. Do you rarely eat anything purple? Pick up some eggplant or red cabbage. Is your diet lacking in orange? Grab some apricots or a butternut squash. This isn't just about fun; it is about ensuring that you are getting a wide variety of phytonutrients to cover all your defensive bases. Your heart loves variety, so give it a full of day—usually around 3:00 PM—when our energy dips and we reach for a candy bar or a soda. This week, I want you to swap that processed sugar for nature's candy. Grab a crisp apple, a handful of grapes, or a juicy peach. You will get the sweet hit you are craving, but instead of a heart-straining sugar crash, you will be getting a steady dose of fiber and antioxidants. It is a small trade that pays massive dividends in your daily energy levels and your long-term heart health.

As you start improves, and you have more "get-up-and-go" in the mornings. These are the outward signs that the internal maintenance crew is doing its job. Your heart is being shielded, your arteries are being smoothed out, and your blood pressure is being supported by the minerals it needs to stay stable. This isn't just about avoiding disease; it is about reaching for a level of vitality that you might have thought was a thing of the past.

Remember, your heart is a living, breathing muscle that is working 24 hours a day to keep you moving. It doesn't ask for much—just the right fuel and a little bit of protection from the elements. By embracing the power of produce, you are giving your heart exactly what it needs to thrive in our modern world. You are taking control of your biological destiny, one bite at a time. The pharmacy of the earth is open for business, and the best part is that the medicine tastes delicious. So, go ahead—fill your plate with color, enjoy the crunch of a fresh vegetable, and know that with every bite, you are building a stronger, healthier, and more vibrant heart. You have the tools, you have the plan, and now you have the power of the plants on your side. Let's keep that heart beating strong for many years to come.

### Reflection Questions

- Is your plate usually colorful, or is it mostly beige and brown? What is one color you can add to your dinner tonight?
- Think back to your childhood. Which vegetables did you actually enjoy eating? How can you bring those back into your weekly meal rotation?
- When you feel a "sugar craving" hit, what is your go-to snack? How can you replace that with a piece of fruit this week to give your heart a break?

By taking the time to answer these questions and implement these simple steps, you are doing more than just following a diet. You are adopting a philosophy of life that prioritizes your most vital organ. Your heart has been with you since before you were born, and it will be with you every step of the way. Give it the vitamins, minerals, and antioxidants it deserves. This is the foundation of a long and healthy life. Keep focused on the goal, and I will see you in the next section where we tackle how to take this heart-healthy lifestyle out into the world.

# Chapter 11
# Dining Out Without the Heartache

So, you've decided to take the reins of your health, you've cleared out the pantry, and you're feeling like a regular fitness pro in your own kitchen. But then the phone rings. It is your best friend, your spouse, or maybe your boss, and they want to go out for a celebratory dinner. Suddenly, a wave of panic hits you. You start thinking about those heavy menus, the smell of deep-fried appetizers a social life and keeping your cardiovascular system in top-notch shape. Well, let me tell you right now: you can have both. You do not have to become a hermit just because you care about your arteries.

Going out to eat is one of life's great pleasures. It is where we celebrate birthdays, close business deals, and catch up with old friends. The problem is that the restaurant industry is built on a very specific set of priorities, and your long-term longevity usually isn't at the top of their list. Chefs want the food to taste amazing so you come back and tell your friends. How do they achieve that? They use the "Big Three" of the professional kitchen: salt, sugar, and fat. They use these ingredients in quantities that would make your jaw drop if you saw them being measured out. But here is the good news. You are the customer. You are the one paying the bill, and that means you are the one in the driver's seat. With a little bit of strategy and a few key phrases, you can navigate any menu like a seasoned pro.

## The Digestive Tax:

## What Happens After the Fork Hits the Plate

Before when you eat a massive, heavy restaurant meal. I like to call this the "Digestive Tax." Most of the time, we think of eating as something that gives us energy, and it does. But the act of digesting food also requires a significant amount of energy and resources from your body. When you sit down to a standard restaurant feast—think a fried appetizer, a buttery steak with a side of loaded mashed potatoes, and a piece of cheesecake—you are essentially declaring a state of emergency for your internal systems.

As soon as that heavy load hits your stomach, your body has to pivot. To break down those fats and proteins, your digestive system requires a massive influx of oxygen-rich blood. Your heart is the engine that has to provide it. It starts beating faster and harder to redirect blood flow away from your brain and your muscles and toward your gut. If you've ever felt that "food coma" or extreme lethargy after a big meal, that is exactly what is happening. Your brain is getting less blood because your stomach is hogging it all. For a healthy person, this is a temporary strain. But if you are already working on improving your heart health, this extra workload is a physical stressor that you want to minimize.

Furthermore, when you consume a high-fat meal, your blood actually your bloodstream. This makes it even harder for your heart to push that blood through the tiny capillaries in your body. It is like trying to pump cold molasses through a straw instead of water. By choosing lighter, heart-smart options when you dine out, you are essentially "lowering the tax." You are allowing your body to get the nutrients it needs without forcing your heart to run a marathon just to process your dinner. You'll leave the restaurant feeling energized and alert instead of bloated and exhausted.

### The Restaurant Survival Guide: 90s Style

In the world of 1990s wellness, we have a very clear set of rules for navigating the "danger zones" of a restaurant menu. These aren't about deprivation; they are about making smarter swaps that don't sacrifice the experience. The first rule of thumb is to become a detective when reading the menu. Words are your clues. If you see terms like "crispy," "breaded," "creamy," "scalloped," or "sautéed in butter," those are red flags for hidden fats. Instead, look for the "Power Words": grilled, broiled, steamed, poached, or roasted. These cooking methods use heat rather than grease to prepare the food, which keeps the flavor in and the unnecessary calories out.

One of the most effective strategies you can use is the "Dressings on the Side" maneuver. This is a classic move for a reason. Most restaurant salads are actually nutritional landmines because they are drenched in half a cup of heavy, oil-based dressing. A the side, you regain control. You can dip the tines of your fork into the dressing before taking a bite of salad. This way, you get the flavor in every mouthful, but you end up using only a fraction of the total amount. It's a simple change that can save you hundreds of calories and dozens of grams of fat without making the salad taste any less delicious.

Another big hurdle is the sheer size of the portions. Have you noticed that restaurant plates seem to be getting bigger every year? In many places, a single "entrée" is actually enough food for two or even three people. Our brains are hardwired to want to finish what is in front of us, especially if we feel like we are "getting our money's worth." But your heart doesn't care about the price-per-ounce; it cares about the volume of work it has to do. A great way to handle this is the "Appetizer as an Entrée" trick. Often, the appetizers are perfectly sized for a single person's meal. Order a shrimp cocktail and a side of steamed vegetables, and you've got a high-protein, low-fat dinner that leaves you feeling satisfied but not stuffed. Alternatively, look for a companion at the table who wants to split a main dish. It saves money, reduces waste, and keeps your heart happy.

### The History of the Drive-Thru: A Global Shift

To understand why dining out has become such a challenge for our health, we have to look back at how our eating habits changed in the mid-20th century. Before the 1950s, eating out was a rare treat for most families. Food was primarily prepared at home, where the cook had total control over the ingredients. But after World War II, the world started moving faster. People wanted convenience, and the "Fast Food Revolution" was born. When the first major burger chains started expanding in the 1950s, they changed the way the entire world viewed a "meal."

Suddenly, food was designed to be consistent, cheap, and fast. To achieve this, companies relied heavily on processed ingredients, high levels of sodium for preservation, and deep-frying for speed. This wasn't just an American phenomenon; these dining habits spread across the globe, bringing a rise in cardiovascular issues to cultures that had previously enjoyed much lower rates of heart disease. We saw a shift from traditional, plant-based diets to the "Western Pattern Diet," which is characterized by high intakes of red meat, sugary desserts, and refined grains. This historical shift is why we now have to be so intentional when we walk into a restaurant. We are fighting against a half-century of culinary engineering designed to appeal to our cravings rather than our longevity.

However, we are also living in a time where the “Wellness Wave” is catching up. More and more restaurants are becoming aware that their customers want healthier options. In the early 90s, we started seeing “Heart Healthy” symbols appearing on menus next to certain items. This was a huge win for the consumer! It showed that the public was demanding better choices. By being an advocate for your own health when you dine out, you are continuing that trend. Every time you ask for a modification or choose the grilled option over the fried one, you are sending a message to the industry that heart health matters. You are part of the solution, not just for yourself, but for the culture at large.

### The Restaurant Script: How to Talk to Your Server

A lot of people feel embarrassed to ask for changes to a dish. They don’t want to be “that person” who is difficult or picky. But let me tell you something: most servers and chefs are happy to accommodate you if you ask politely. They want you to enjoy your meal! The key is to have a “script” ready so you can make your requests confidently and clearly. You aren’t being a nuisance; you are being a responsible owner of your body. Here are a few ways to phrase your requests that are polite and effective:

- **The Butter Barrier:** “I’d love the grilled salmon, but could you ask the chef to prepare it without any extra butter or oil? A little lemon and herbs would be great instead."

- **The Vegetable Swap:** "I see the steak comes with fries. Is it possible to swap those out for a double portion of the steamed broccoli?"

- **The Dressing Detail:** "I'll have the garden salad, please, but could I get the balsamic dressing on the side? Also, could we skip the croutons and cheese?"

- **The Preparation Probe:** "Is the chicken in this dish breaded and fried, or is it grilled? If it's fried, could I have a grilled chicken breast substituted instead?"

When you use these scripts, you are taking the guesswork out of the meal. You are ensuring that what arrives at your table aligns with your goals. Most of the time, the kitchen is already prepping these ingredients, so a simple swap isn't a big deal for them at all. In fact, many high-end chefs appreciate a customer who cares about the quality and preparation of their food. Don't be afraid to speak up. Your health is worth a thirty-second conversation with your waiter.

### Strategic Maneuvers: The Pre-Meal Water Trick

One of the biggest traps of dining out happens before the food even arrives. You sit down, you're hungry, and the server immediately drops a basket of warm bread or a bowl of salty chips on the table. Before you know it, you've consumed 300 calories of refined flour and butter, and you haven't even looked at the menu yet. This is where "The Pre-Meal Water Trick" comes into play. As soon as you sit down, ask for a large glass of water with lemon. Drink the entire glass before you even touch the bread basket. This does two things: it hydrates you (which often reduces the feeling of false hunger) and it physically takes up space in your stomach.

When your stomach is partially full of water, the "satiety signals" that tell your brain you are full will fire much sooner. You'll find it much easier to have just one small piece of bread—or skip it entirely—because you aren't operating on a completely empty tank. Additionally, choosing water as your primary beverage throughout the meal is a major win for your heart. Alcohol and sugary sodas add "empty" calories and can actually increase your appetite, making you more likely to overeat. Water, on the other hand, aids digestion and keeps your blood volume stable. If you want something with a bit more zing, try sparkling water with a splash of lime. It feels like a "fancy" drink but has zero negative impact on your cardiovascular goals.

### Action Plan: Dining with Confidence

Now that we've covered the "why" and the "how," it is time to put these strategies into a concrete plan of action. You don't have to do everything at once, but choosing one or two of these habits to implement next time you go out will make a world of difference. Here is your step-by-step guide to a heart-smart night on the town.

1. **Decisions Made While You're Hungry**

When the waiter is standing over you and everyone else is ordering the bacon-wrapped whatever, it is very easy to cave to the pressure. You can avoid this by looking up the menu online before you even leave the house. Most restaurants have their menus posted on their websites or on social media. Take five minutes to look through the options while you are calm and not hungry. Identify two or three "safe" choices that look delicious and fit your heart-smartre getting. This removes the "decision fatigue" and the temptation to stray from your plan.

**2. The Half-Plate Rule**

This is perhaps the most powerful tool in your restaurant arsenal. As we discussed, full, use the "Doggy Bag Strategy." As soon as your meal arrives, ask the server for a "to-go" your plate, and you have a delicious lunch for tomorrow already prepared. By getting the extra food off your plate and out of sight, you remove the visual cue to keep eating. You'll find that you are perfectly satisfied with the half-portion, and your heart won't have to pay that heavy "Digestive Tax."

**3. Be Your Own Advocate**

This week, I want you to practice making at least one modification to a restaurant order. It doesn't have to be a big deal. It could be as simple as asking for your potato to be plain instead of loaded, or asking for steamed vegetables instead of fries. The goal is to get comfortable with the idea that you have a say in how your food is prepared. Remember, you aren't being "difficult." You are being proactive about your health. The more you do it, the more natural it will feel. You'll eventually realize that most restaurants are happy to help you eat better, and the food often tastes fresher and more vibrant when it isn't covered in heavy sauces.

## Common Pitfalls to Avoid

Even the most well-intentioned diner can get tripped up by a few common mistakes. One of the most frequent is the "Salad Seduction." Just because a dish is called a "salad" doesn't mean it is healthy. Many chain restaurants offer salads that are loaded with fried chicken strips, candied walnuts, three types of cheese, and a creamy ranch dressing. These can easily clock in at over 1,000 calories and massive amounts of saturated fat. Always that are primarily greens and fresh vegetables, with lean proteins like grilled chicken or chickpeas.

Another mistake is the "I'm Paying for It" mentality. We often feel like if we don't clean our plates, we are wasting money. But think about it this way: if you eat food that your body doesn't need, you are still "wasting" it—you're just using your body as a trash can. The money is spent whether you eat the food or not. If you eat past the point of fullness, you are paying a "tax" in the form of stress on your heart and sluggishness in your day. It is far better to leave a few bites on the plate or take them home for later than to force your heart to process excess calories that provide no benefit.

Finally, watch out for the "Healthy Halo." This happens when we think that because we ordered a healthy main dish, we can "afford" to have a high-fat appetizer or a sugary dessert. "I had the grilled fish, so I can have the mud pie!" While balance is important, those high-fat add-ons can quickly undo all the good work of your main choice. If you really want a treat, try sharing one dessert with the whole table. Everyone gets a couple of bites of the sweetness, but no one ends up with a massive dose of sugar and fat that leaves their heart pounding.

## Reflecting on Your Progress

As you start to navigate the world of dining out with these new tools, take a moment to notice how your experience changes. You might find that you actually enjoy the food more when you can taste the actual ingredients instead of just the salt and fat. You might notice that you have more energy for the conversation at the table because your body isn't working overtime to digest a massive meal. These are the "hidden" benefits of heart-smart dining. It isn't just about your cholesterol numbers; it is about the quality of your life in the moments that matter most.

Think about your next scheduled meal out. What is the name of the restaurant? Have you looked at their menu yet? Which of the "scripts" we talked about today could you use to make that meal a little bit better for your heart? By asking these questions and making a plan, you are taking ownership of your health in a very real, practical way. You are proving that you don't have to sacrifice your joy to have a strong, healthy heart. You are becoming a person who can enjoy the best of both your new "Restaurant Survival Guide" in hand, you are ready to walk into any bistro, cafe, or steakhouse with confidence. You know the "Digestive Tax" and how to avoid it. You know the "Power Words" to look for and the "Red Flags" to avoid. You are equipped with the scripts you need to be your own advocate. Most importantly, you are beginning to see that every meal is an opportunity to support your heart and build a future of vitality and health. So go ahead, make that reservation. Your heart is ready for a night out, and now, you are too.

**You Must Be Your Own Health Advocate**

1. Heavy meals create a "Digestive Tax" that forces the heart to work harder.
2. Use the "Half-Plate Rule" to manage massive portions and prevent overeating.
3. Always ask for dressings and sauces on the side to maintain control.
4. Researching the menu before you arrive eliminates impulsive, unhealthy choices.

By following these simple strategies, you are ensuring that your social life and your heart health can coexist beautifully. You are learning that a healthy lifestyle isn't about saying "no" to everything; it's about saying "yes" to the right things in the right ways. Keep that momentum going, and remember that every smart choice you make at the dinner table is a victory for your heart. You are doing the work, you are seeing the results, and you are building a life that you can truly enjoy for a long, long time. Let's keep moving forward toward that goal of peak vitality.

# Chapter 12
## Aerobics:
## The Heart of the Workout

Are you ready to feel the fire? Say, you want to live longer? How about taking steps to improve your body through sweat, movement, and a real understanding of how your internal engine handles the load? Well, you have come to the right place. We have talked about what you put into your body, and we have talked about how to navigate the social pressures of the dinner table. Now, it is time to get those sneakers laced up, because we are about to jump into the most vital part of your fitness journey: aerobics. This is where the rubber meets the road, or more accurately, where your feet meet the pavement and your heart meets its potential.

The words "aerobic activity" mean you are training your entire cardiovascular system to become more efficient, more resilient, and more powerful. It is not just about burning calories or fitting into those slim-cut jeans you bought back in '88. It is about making your heart a champion. When you commit to a regular aerobic routine, you are essentially giving your body a tune-up that affects every single cell from your head to your toes. The energy you feel, the clarity of your thoughts, and the strength of your pulse all depend on this oxygen-rich process.

## The Physics of the Pump: Stroke Volume

Let's get into some Anatomy 101. To understand why aerobics is the gold standard for heart health, you have to understand a concept called **Stroke Volume**. Think of your heart as a pump in a high-tech factory. Stroke volume is the amount of blood that the left ventricle of your heart ejects with every single contraction. It is a measurement of how much work your heart can do in one go. Now, why does this matter to you? Because a heart that is trained through aerobic exercise is a heart that has a higher stroke volume. It becomes more efficient. It doesn on the couch, your heart might beat 70 or 80 times per minute to keep your blood moving. But for a highly trained aerobic athlete, that resting heart rate might drop to 50 or even 40 beats per minute. Their heart is so strong that it can move the same amount of blood—or more—with far fewer contractions. Over the course of a lifetime, that adds up to millions of fewer beats. You are essentially saving the wear and tear on your cardiac muscle while simultaneously making it stronger. Aerobic exercise causes the chambers of the heart, particularly the left ventricle, to slightly enlarge and the muscle walls to become more pliable and strong. This allows the heart to fill with more blood and then snap shut with more force, sending a larger volume of oxygenated blood out to your muscles.

This process also improves your **Cardiac Output**, which is the total amount of blood your heart pumps in one minute. When you are exercising at a high intensity, your body's demand for oxygen skyrockets. Your muscles are hungry, and they need fuel to keep moving. A heart with a high stroke volume can meet this demand without hitting its redline too quickly. You'll find that you can walk faster, climb stairs easier, and play with your kids or grandkids without feeling like you are gasping for air. This is the physiological reality of "getting in shape." You aren't just losing weight; you are re-engineering your internal plumbing to handle more pressure with less stress.

**The 1960s Spark:**

**Dr. Kenneth Cooper and a crime scene!**

The common wisdom of the day suggested that heavy exercise was a strain that should be avoided as you aged. But all of that changed in 1968 when a physician named Dr. Kenneth Cooper published a book simply titled *Aerobics*. Dr. Cooper was a flight surgeon for the Air Force, and he noticed that some pilots who were in "good shape" by traditional standards actually had terrible cardiovascular endurance. He developed a system of points and exercises designed to improve the body's ability to use oxygen.

Dr. Cooper's research showed that the real key to longevity wasn't big muscles or being able to lift heavy weights; it was the health of the lungs and the heart. He proved that regular, sustained activity—like running, swimming, or cycling—could prevent heart disease and increase life expectancy. His book sold millions of copies and launched a global fitness revolution. Suddenly, people realized that they weren't fragile. They realized that the human body was designed to move. By the time we hit the late 1970s and 80s, this movement had evolved into the high-energy, neon-colored world of aerobic dance classes and step routines that we know today.

We owe a lot to that 1968 milestone. It shifted the focus of medicine from treatment to prevention. It gave us the tools to take our health into our own hands. Before Dr. Cooper, if you had a heart problem, the doctor might prescribe "bed rest." Today, we know that is the worst thing you can do! The best medicine for a weak heart is carefully managed movement. We have moved from a sedentary culture to one that prizes vitality, and it all started with the realization that our hearts thrive when we challenge them. When you step onto that treadmill or join that low-impact class, you are participating in a legacy of health that has transformed how we understand the human body.

### The 3-Phase Workout: Your 30-Minute Roadmap

Now that you know the history and the science, let's get down to business. You don't need to spend hours in the gym to see massive improvements in your heart health. In fact, a focused, 30-minute session is all it takes to get into the zone. The key is structure. You can't just jump from a dead stop into a full-speed sprint. That is a recipe for injury and unnecessary cardiac stress. We use a 3-phase approach that ensures your heart is prepared, challenged, and then safely brought back to a resting state. This is the ultimate wellness strategy for the modern era.

### Phase 1: The Warmup (5 Minutes)

Think of your body like a car on a cold winter morning. You wouldn't start the engine and immediately floor it onto the highway, would you? Of course not. You let the oil circulate and the engine block warm up. Your body is the same way. During the warmup, you are gradually increasing your heart rate and body temperature. This sends a signal to your blood vessels to dilate, allowing for better blood flow. It also lubricates your in place, do some light arm circles, or take a very slow stroll around the living room. The goal is not to get out of breath. You should still be able to sing a song or hold a full conversation without any effort. You are simply waking up the system. You might start to feel a little bit of warmth in your skin, and that is a good sign. It means the blood is moving from your internal organs out to your extremities, preparing you for the "Peak" phase.

### Phase 2: The Peak – Entering the Target Zone (20 Minutes)

This is the core of the workout. This is where the magic happens. To get the aerobic benefits we've been talking about, you need to stay in your **Target Heart Rate Zone** for at least 20 minutes. This is the level of intensity where your heart is beating fast enough to build strength, but not so fast that you are straining yourself. For most people, this means your heart rate should be between 60% and 80% of your maximum heart rate. A quick way to estimate your maximum heart rate is to subtract your age from 220. So, if you are 50 years old, your estimated max is 170 beats per minute. Your target zone would be roughly between 102 and 136 beats per minute.

During these 20 minutes, you want to maintain a steady level of activity. This could be a brisk walk, a low-impact aerobic video, or even some vigorous gardening. The "Talk Test" is your best friend here. You should be working hard enough that you can speak in short sentences, but you shouldn't be able to belt out a Broadway show tune. If you can't speak at all, you are working too hard—slow down! If you can talk for minutes without pausing for air, you need to pick up the pace. This 20-minute block is where you are training that stroke volume and teaching your heart to be a more efficient pump.

### Phase 3: The Cooldown (5 Minutes)

Never, ever skip the cooldown. This is one of the most common mistakes people make. When you are exercising hard, your leg muscles are acting as "second hearts," helping to pump blood back up to your chest. If you stop abruptly, that blood can pool in your legs, which can lead to dizziness, fainting, or even an irregular heartbeat. The cooldown allows your heart rate to drop slowly and your blood pressure to stabilize.

For the final 5 minutes, simply slow your pace. If you were walking briskly, slow down to a leisurely stroll. Do some gentle stretching—nothing bouncy or intense. Focus on deep, rhythmic breathing. You want to feel your pulse gradually return to normal. By the time you finish, you should feel refreshed and energized, not exhausted or "wiped out." A good workout should give you energy for the rest of your day, not take it away.

### The Art of Pulse Monitoring

How do you know if you are actually in the zone? In our era, we don't need fancy computers strapped to our wrists to know what's going on inside. You have two built-in sensors right on your body: the radial pulse on your wrist and the carotid pulse on your neck. Learning to check your pulse manually is a vital skill for anyone serious about heart health. It gives you immediate, real-time feedback on how your engine is performing.

To check your radial pulse, turn your palm up. Use the tips of your index and middle fingers (never your thumb, as it has its own pulse!) and place them on the thumb side of your wrist, just below the base of the hand. Press lightly until you feel the rhythmic "thump." To check your carotid pulse, place your fingers on the side of your neck, just under the jawline. Be careful not to press too hard on the neck, as this can actually slow the heart rate down. Once you find the beat, look at a watch with a second hand. Count the beats for 10 seconds, then multiply that number by 6. That is your heart rate in beats per minute.

I recommend checking your pulse about halfway through your "Peak" phase. If your 10-second count is 20 beats, your heart rate is 120. If that fits within your target zone, keep going! If it's too high, take it down a notch. If it's too low, move those arms and legs a little faster. You should also check your pulse immediately after your cooldown. This is your "recovery heart rate." Over time, as your heart gets stronger, you will notice that your heart rate returns to its resting level much faster after exercise. That is a clear, measurable sign that your stroke volume is improving and your heart is becoming a world-class athlete.

### Low-Impact, High-Reward: Movement for Everyone

A common misconception is that you have to be a marathon runner or a high-jumping gymnast to get the benefits of aerobics. That couldn't be further from the truth. In fact, for many of us, **low-impact aerobics** is actually better for long-term health. Low-impact means that one foot is always on the ground. There is no jumping, no pounding, and no jarring of the joints. This protects your knees, hips, and lower back while still giving your heart the challenge it needs.

Think about activities like brisk walking, swimming, or using a stationary bike. These are all low-impact, but they are incredibly effective at improving cardiovascular health. You can even do an aerobic routine right in your living room while watching the evening news. Side-to-side steps, grapevines, and knee lifts are all fantastic ways to get the heart rate up without hurting your body. The goal is consistency, not intensity. A 30-minute walk every day is infinitely better for your heart than a five-mile run once a month. Your heart thrives on the regular, predictable rhythm of daily movement.

If you are just starting out, don't feel like you have to hit the full 20 minutes in the target zone right away. It is perfectly fine to start with 5 or 10 minutes and build up as you feel stronger. The most important thing is that you are moving. Every step you take is a vote for a longer, healthier life. You are training your body to be efficient, and that training takes time. Be patient with yourself, but be persistent. The "runner's high"—that feeling of euphoria and accomplishment—isn't reserved for people in spandex; it's available to anyone who gets their blood pumping and their oxygen flowing.

### The Power of the Playlist

Let's talk about the mental side of the workout. Sometimes, the hardest part of aerobics isn't the physical effort; it's the boredom. Staring at a wall while you march in place can make five minutes feel like fifty. That is why music is your secret weapon. The right beat can actually synchronize with your heart rate and make the exercise feel easier. It distracts your brain from the sensation of effort and allows you to stay in the zone longer.

In the 90s, we know the power of a high-energy soundtrack. When you hear a song with a steady, driving rhythm, your body naturally wants to move in time with it. I want you to create a "Heart-Smart Playlist." Look for songs that have about 120 to 140 beats per minute for your peak phase. For your warmup and cooldown, choose something slower and more relaxing. When the music is right, you aren't just "working out"—you are dancing, you are grooving, and you are having fun. When exercise is fun, you are much more likely to keep doing it. So, turn up the volume and let the music carry you through those 30 minutes. Your heart will thank you for the party!

### Common Mistakes to Avoid

Even with the best intentions, it is easy to fall. I know you're busy, and you want to get the workout over with, but those five minutes of preparation are essential. Jumping straight into intense exercise can cause a sudden spike in blood pressure and put unnecessary strain on your heart valves. It's like trying to stretch a cold rubber band; it's much more likely to snap. Take the time to get warm.

Another mistake is **stopping abruptly**. We talked about blood pooling in the legs, but there is also a psychological component. Stopping suddenly can leave you feeling dizzy and nauseous, which creates a negative association with exercise. You want to finish your workout feeling like a million bucks, not like you're about to keel over. The cooldown is your "victory lap." Use it to celebrate the work you just did.

Finally, watch out for the **"No Pain, No Gain"** trap. This was a popular slogan for a while, but it is actually quite dangerous when it comes to heart health. Aerobic exercise should be challenging, yes, but it should never be painful. If you feel chest pain, extreme shortness of breath, or lightheadedness, stop immediately. Those are red flags from your heart telling you that something is wrong. A healthy workout should make you breathe deeply and sweat, but it shouldn't cause agony. Listen to your body; it's the only one you've got, and it knows its limits better than any book or trainer.

**The History of the Step: Innovation in the Living Room**

As we look at how aerobics has evolved, we have to mention the pro Gin Miller, who was looking for a way to rehabilitate a knee injury. She discovered that stepping up and down on a milk crate gave her a great cardiovascular workout without the impact of running. This led to the creation of the plastic "Step" platforms that you see in gyms everywhere today.

The beauty of the step workout was its simplicity and by just walking on a flat surface. It also toned the large muscles of the legs—the glutes, quads, and hamstrings—which are the primary drivers of your metabolic furnace. The more muscle you engage, the more oxygen your heart has to deliver own homes. It democratized fitness, making heart health accessible to anyone with a little bit of floor space and a sturdy platform.

This period in history was all about empowerment. We were learning that we didn't need to be elite athletes to have elite-level heart health. The tools were becoming simpler, the information was becoming clearer, and the results were undeniable. People who had never exercised a day in their lives were finding joy in movement. That same spirit of accessibility is what I want you to embrace today. You don't need fancy equipment. You just need the willingness to move and the knowledge of how to do it safely.

### Action Plan: Your First 30-Minute Session

It is time to take everything we have discussed and turn it into action. Reading about aerobics is great, but the benefits only come when you actually get your heart rate up. This week, I want you to commit to three sessions of the 30-minute cardio routine. You don't have to go to a gym; you can do this right where you are. Here is your step-by-step guide to success.

1. **Set the Stage:** Put on your favorite upbeat music. Choose songs that make you want to tap your toes and move your shoulders. Wear comfortable shoes with good support and clothes that allow you to move freely. Have a bottle of water nearby.

2. **The 5-Minute Warmup:** Start by marching in place. Lift your knees gently and swing your arms in a natural rhythm. After two minutes, add some side-to-side steps. Reach your arms out to the sides and then overhead. By the end of the five minutes, you should feel warm and your breathing should be slightly deeper.

3. **The 20-Minute Target Zone:** Pick up the pace. You can do a brisk walk around your neighborhood, follow a low-impact aerobic video, or continue your

marching with more intensity—lifting your knees higher and pumping your arms more vigorously. About ten minutes in, check your pulse. Are you in your target zone? Adjust your intensity as needed. Remember the "Talk Test"—you should be able to speak, but not sing.

4. **The 5-Minute Cooldown:** Slow down your movements. Walk at a very easy pace. Let your arms hang loosely at your sides. Take deep, slow breaths in through your nose and out through your mouth. Do some gentle stretches for your calves and thighs, holding each stretch for 15-20 seconds without bouncing.

5. **Record Your Progress:** After your cooldown, take your pulse one last time. Write it down in a notebook along with your resting heart rate from earlier in the day. Note how you felt during the workout. Did you have a "runner's high"? Did you feel strong? Tracking these small victories is what keeps you motivated for the long haul.

### The Long-Term Vision: Consistency Over Intensity

As you begin this journey, remember that you are playing the "long game." A single 30-minute workout is a great start, but the real transformation of your heart happens over months and years of consistent effort. You are building a habit that will serve you for the rest of your life. There will be days when you don't feel like moving, and that's okay. On those days, tell yourself you'll just do the 5-minute warmup. Usually, once you get started, you'll find the energy to finish the whole session. And if you don't? At least you moved for five minutes, and that still counts!

Aerobics is the heart of the workout because it directly addresses the most important muscle in your body. It is the foundation upon which all other fitness is built. When your heart is strong, everything else becomes easier. You'll have more energy for your hobbies, more stamina for your work, and a more positive outlook on life. You are taking ownership of your vitality. You are choosing to be active rather than passive in your own health. This is a powerful shift in mindset that will ripple out into every area of your life.

So, what are you waiting for? The music is playing, your sneakers are ready, and your heart is waiting for the challenge. You have the science of stroke volume to guide you, the history of the aerobics movement to inspire you, and a clear 30-minute plan to follow. You are no longer guessing at what works; you have the roadmap to success. Let's get that heart rate up and start building the strong, resilient, healthy future you deserve. Your heart is the engine of your life, and today, you are the lead mechanic. Let's make it purr!

## Reflecting on the Rhythm

As you finish this chapter, take a moment to think about your relationship with movement. For many of us, exercise has felt like a chore or a punishment for what we ate. I want you to flip that script. Aerobic exercise is a gift you give to your heart. It is an opportunity to feel alive, to breathe deeply, and to celebrate what your body can do. How can you make your 30-minute cardio sessions the best part of your day? Maybe it's the time you listen to your favorite podcast, or maybe it's a time for quiet reflection while you walk through a local park.

Think about the "runner's high." Have you ever felt that rush of endorphins after a period of physical activity? That is your body's natural way of rewarding you for taking care of your heart. It's a sense of accomplishment and peace that can't be bought in a bottle. As you move through your action plan this week, pay attention to that feeling. Let it be your motivation. You aren't just working out to reach a number on a scale; you are working out to feel that sense of peak vitality.

Your heart is an incredible organ. It works for you every second of every day without you even having to think about it. By engaging in regular aerobics, you are finally giving something back to it. You are providing the challenge it needs to stay strong and the care it needs to last a lifetime. You are the boss of your body, and the choices you make today will determine the quality of your tomorrows. Keep moving, keep breathing, and keep listening to the steady, strong rhythm of your heart. It's telling you that you're doing a great job.

**Key Takeaways for a Stronger Heart**

- **Aerobics is Oxygen Power:** Activities that use oxygen to fuel movement are the best way to strengthen the cardiovascular system.
- **Stroke Volume is Efficiency:** Training your heart allows it to pump more blood with each beat, reducing the total workload on the muscle.
- **The 3-Phase Rule:** Always include a warmup, a peak phase in the target zone, and a cooldown to ensure safety and effectiveness.

- **Monitor Your Progress:** Use the 10-second pulse check to stay in your target zone and track your recovery heart rate over time.

- **Low-Impact works:** You don't need to pound your joints to get a world-class heart workout. Brisk walking and steady movement are highly effective.

- **Music is Fuel:** Use high-energy songs to keep your motivation high and your rhythm steady during your 20-minute peak phase.

By following these principles, you are making heart health a practical, enjoyable part of your daily life. You are moving away from the "all or nothing" mentality and toward a sustainable lifestyle of vitality. The path to a healthier heart isn't a sprint; it's a steady, rhythmic walk toward a better version of yourself. You have the tools, you have the plan, and you have the heart to make it happen. Let's keep that momentum going as we move into the next phase of our journey together. You are doing amazing work, and your heart knows it!

# Chapter 13
## Walking for Life: The Simplest Secret

Think about the last time you saw someone walking down the street with a purpose. Maybe they had their elbows tucked in, their arms swinging like a metronome, and a look of pure determination on their face. You might have chuckled a bit at the sight, but let me tell you, that person was onto something big. They weren't just getting from point A to point B; they were engaging in one of the most effective, accessible, and sustainable ways to keep their pulse strong and their body lean. You don't need a high-priced club membership or a complicated piece of machinery that takes up half your guest bedroom to save your life. You just need the two feet you were born with and a little bit of sidewalk.

Walking is the original human exercise. Before we had stationary bikes or cross-trainers, we were a species on the move. We are built for it. Every bone, every tendon, and every muscle of movement is a quiet tragedy for the human pump. When we stop moving, our circulation slows down, our muscles lose their tone, and our hearts have to work much harder just to do the basics. But the good news is that you can reverse this trend starting of you are thinking. "Walking? That's too easy! I need to be sweating buckets and gasping for air to get a real workout." Well, I'm here to set the record straight. Walking is a powerhouse of cardiovascular health. It provides a steady, rhythmic challenge that builds endurance without the jarring impact that can ruin your knees and ankles. It's the perfect entry point for someone who hasn't exercised in years, and it remains a foundational habit for the most elite athletes. When you walk, you are engaging in a dialogue with your body, telling it that you are ready for life, ready for energy, and ready for longevity. Let's get into why this simple act is actually a sophisticated piece of biological engineering.

## The Second Heart: Your Calf Muscles

To understand the genius of walking, we have to look below the waist. In medical circles, the calf muscles are often called the **venous pumps** or even the "second heart." This isn't just a colorful nickname; it describes a critical physiological function. Your heart is great at pushing blood out to your extremities through your arteries, but getting that blood all the way back up from your toes against the relentless pull of gravity is a much harder job. This is where your legs come into play.

The veins in your legs have one-way valves that allow blood to move upward but prevent it from flowing back down. This squeezing action acts like a secondary pump, boosting the blood back toward your chest. When you walk, you are literally assisting your heart in its daily chores. By using your legs, you reduce the workload on your cardiac muscle, allowing it to operate more efficiently. It's like having a teammate who handles the heavy lifting so you can focus on the strategy.

When we stay sedentary for too long, this pump stays idle. Blood can begin to pool in the lower legs, which is why your ankles might feel swollen after a long flight or a day spent sitting at a desk. Over time, these sluggish pumps kick into gear. The oxygen-depleted blood is sent back to the lungs to be refreshed, and the cycle of life continues at a much more vigorous pace. This is why a simple stroll can make you feel so much more alert.

Furthermore, this "second heart" mechanism helps regulate your blood pressure. By facilitating the return of blood to the heart, the venous pump ensures a steady stroke volume. As we learned previously, a consistent and efficient stroke volume is the hallmark of a healthy cardiovascular system. When you walk at a brisk pace, you are training these leg muscles to be reliable partners for your heart. You aren't just "toning your legs"; you are optimizing your entire circulatory network. It's a beautiful system of cooperation that only requires you to put one foot in front of the other.

### Mastering the Power Walk

Now, we aren't talking about a leisurely window-shopping stroll here. If you want to see real changes in your fitness, you need to adopt a specific technique. In the wellness circles of the 90s, we call this the **Power Walk**. This is a purposeful, high-energy version of walking that maximizes your caloric burn and gets your heart rate into that vital target zone. It's about form, rhythm, and intention. If you do it right, you'll feel the difference in every fiber of your being.

The first thing to focus on is your posture. Stand tall, as if there's a string pulling the top of your head toward the sky. Keep your chin up and your eyes looking about twenty feet ahead of you. This opens up your chest and allows your lungs to expand fully. If you slouch or look at your feet, you're compressing your diaphragm, which makes it harder for your heart to get the oxygen it needs. A tall posture also engages your core muscles, providing a stable base for your legs to move. Think of yourself as a finely tuned machine, streamlined and ready for action.

Next, let's talk about the **arm swing**. This is the secret ingredient of the power walk. Your arms should be bent at a ninety-degree angle, and they should swing naturally from the shoulders, not the elbows. As you step forward with your left foot, your right arm should swing forward, and vice versa. Don't let your hands cross the midline of your body; keep them moving in a straight forward-and-back motion. The faster you swing your arms, the faster your legs will follow. It's a neurological connection that you can use to your advantage. By involving your upper body, you're turning a leg exercise into a full-body workout, burning more calories and putting a greater demand on your heart.

The third element is the **heel-to-toe roll**. This is the proper way to strike the ground. You want your heel to hit first, then roll the weight through the arch of your foot, and finally with your toes also gives your calves that extra squeeze we talked about, maximizing the venous pump effect. It should feel like a smooth, continuous flow of energy from the ground up through your body.

Finally, you need to maintain a **purposeful pace**. You should be moving fast enough that you feel your heart rate climb and your breathing become more rhythmic. You might even break a light sweat. A good rule of thumb is the "urgent" pace—walk as if you're five minutes late for a very important meeting with a very important person. You aren't running, but you certainly aren't dawdling. This level of intensity is where the cardiovascular benefits really start to accumulate. When you combine these four elements—posture, arm swing, heel-to-toe roll, and pace—you transform a simple walk into a potent health-building tool.

## The Evolutionary Mismatch

Why is walking so effective for us? To find the answer, we have to look back at the history of the human race. For hundreds of thousands of years, our ancestors were hunter-gatherers. They didn't have cars, bikes, or even horses for the vast majority of our history. If they wanted to find food, water, or a new place to sleep, they had to walk. Anthropologists tell us that early humans likely covered ten to fifteen miles a day on foot. Our bodies evolved under these conditions. Our hearts, our lungs, and our metabolic systems are all optimized for frequent, low-to-moderate intensity movement over long periods.

This is why the modern sedentary lifestyle feels so "unnatural" to our biology. In the span of just a few generations, we've gone from walking all day to sitting for fourteen or sixteen hours a day. This is what scientists call an **evolutionary mismatch**. Our genes are still programmed for the savanna, but our lives are lived in cubicles and armchairs. When we don't move, our bodies get confused. They start storing extra fat because they think we're preparing for a famine that never comes. Our hearts become less efficient because they aren't being challenged to pump blood against the resistance of movement. The "diseases of civilization"—heart disease, type 2 diabetes, and hypertension—are often the direct result of this mismatch.

Walking is the simplest way to bridge this gap. When you go for a thirty-minute walk, you are giving your body exactly what it expects. You are speaking the language that your DNA understands. This is why walking has such a profound effect on our mental state as well. Have you ever noticed that your best ideas come to you when you're out for a stroll? Or how a bad mood seems to evaporate after a mile or two? That's because movement triggers the release of endorphins and improves blood flow to the brain. It's how we were meant to function. We aren't designed to be still; we are designed to be in motion.

Understanding this history should give you a sense of empowerment. You aren't fighting against your body when you exercise; you are returning it to its natural state. You don't have to "become" a fitness person; you just have to reclaim the heritage that is already inside you. Every step you take is a connection to the thousands of generations that came before you. It's a way of honoring the incredible machinery that you've inherited. When you look at it that way, a walk isn't just a chore on your to-do list; it's a vital act of self-care that aligns your modern life with your ancient biological needs.

## The Magic of Intervals

If you want to take your walking routine to the next level, I have a secret weapon for you: **Interval Walking**. This is a technique where you alternate between your normal power-walking pace and a shorter burst of "as-fast-as-you-can" walking. This simple change can dramatically increase the cardiovascular benefits of your workout and help you break through any fitness plateaus you might be hitting. It's a way of "tricking" your heart into working harder for short periods, which builds strength and resilience much faster than a steady pace alone.

Here is how it works. After your five-minute warmup at a normal pace, pick up the speed to your purposeful power walk for about three minutes. Then, for one minute, walk as fast as you possibly can without breaking into a jog. Pump those arms, push off those toes, and really give it your all. You should be breathing hard by the end of that minute. After the fast burst, return to your power-walking pace for another three minutes to let your heart rate recover slightly. Repeat this cycle four or five times during your workout before finishing with a five-minute cooldown.

This “fast-slow” pattern is incredibly effective for a few reasons. First, it increases your **aerobic capacity**. By pushing your heart rate higher during the fast intervals, you’re teaching your heart to handle more stress. Second, it keeps your metabolism elevated for hours after you finish your walk. This is known as the “afterburn” effect. Your body has to work harder to return to its resting state after an interval session, which means you’re burning more calories even while you’re sitting on the couch later that evening. Finally, intervals prevent boredom. The workout goes by much faster when you’re focused on the clock and your changing pace.

Interval walking is also a great way to measure your progress. In the beginning, that one-minute burst might feel like a marathon. But after a few weeks, you’ll find that you can go faster and recover more quickly. You’ll notice that your “recovery heart rate”—how fast your pulse returns to normal after the burst—is dropping. That is a clear, objective sign that your heart is getting stronger. It’s the kind of tangible evidence that keeps you motivated to lace up your shoes day after day. You are literally watching yourself become more fit, one interval at a time.

## Every Step Counts

While a dedicated thirty-minute walk is the gold standard, I want to introduce you to the concept of **incidental steps**. These are the steps you take during the normal course of your day that aren't part of a formal "workout." In our modern world, we've become experts at avoiding these steps. We look for the closest parking spot, we take the elevator instead of the stairs, and we use the remote control so we don't have to stand up to change the channel. But these tiny moments of movement add up to something significant over the course of a week, a month, and a year.

I want you to start looking at your environment as a hidden gymnasium. Every staircase is a chance to build heart strength. Every long hallway is an opportunity to engage your venous pumps. When you choose the "harder" way to move through your day, you are making a deposit into your health account. These incidental steps might not get your heart rate into the target zone for twenty minutes, but they keep your metabolism humming and prevent your circulation from stagnating. They are the "background radiation" of a healthy life.

Think about your daily routine. Could you park at the very back of the lot when you go to the grocery store? That might add five hundred steps to your day. Could you use the restroom on a different floor at work and take the stairs to get there? That's another few hundred steps plus a vertical challenge for your heart. Could you pace around the room while you're on the phone instead of sitting in your chair? Over a twenty-minute conversation, you could easily cover half a mile.

The beauty of tracking these steps—perhaps with one of those simple clip-on pedometers that are becoming so popular—is that it turns your day into a game. You start to see how everything connects. You realize that a busy day of errands is actually a great workout in disguise. It takes the pressure off "the workout" and makes health a continuous process. When you combine these incidental steps with your daily power walk, you become a movement machine. You are constantly feeding your heart the activity it craves, and the results will show in your energy levels, your weight, and your overall sense of well-being.

### Your Action Plan: Step by Step

It's time to take this knowledge and put it onto the pavement. Reading about walking is the first step, but the real magic happens when your soles hit the dirt. I want to give you a clear, no-excuses plan to make walking a permanent part of your heart-healthy lifestyle. This isn't about a temporary "fix"; it's about a new way of living that will serve you for decades to come. Let's break it down into three simple, actionable goals for this week.

1. **Commit to a daily 30-minute walk.** This is your non-negotiable appointment with yourself. It doesn't matter if you do it in the morning, during your lunch break, or after dinner. Just get it done. Use the power-walk technique we discussed: stand tall, swing those arms, and roll from heel to toe. If thirty minutes feels like too much at first, start with fifteen and add a minute every day. The goal is consistency. Your heart doesn't care how fast you go in the beginning; it just cares that you show up.

2. **Find a walking partner.** Everything is easier when you have a buddy. Find a friend, a spouse, or a neighbor who also wants to improve their health. Having someone waiting for you at the corner at 7:00 AM is the best accountability tool in the world. It's much harder to hit the snooze button when you know you're letting someone else down. Plus, walking is a great time for social connection. You can catch up on each other's lives while you're both doing something great for your hearts. If you can't find a human partner, a dog is an excellent substitute—they are always ready for a walk!

3. **Increase your 'incidental' steps.** Make a conscious effort to move more during your "non-exercise" hours. Park at the back of the lot. Take the stairs. Stand up and stretch every hour. These small actions keep your venous pumps active and your circulation flowing throughout the day. Try to find three new ways each day to add extra steps to your routine. It's like finding "free" health benefits hidden in your normal schedule.

As you start this plan, pay attention to how you feel. Notice the clarity in your mind after a walk. Notice how much better you sleep at night. Notice the sense of accomplishment you feel when you check that walk off your list. These are the real rewards of a heart-healthy lifestyle. You aren't just doing this to avoid a problem; you're doing it to gain a better life. You are taking charge of your most vital organ and giving it the support it needs to keep you going strong.

## Common Pitfalls and How to Avoid Them

Even a simple habit like walking can have its challenges. One of the biggest mistakes people make is **walking too slowly**. If you're just ambling along at the same pace you use to walk from the bed to the bathroom, you aren't going to see much cardiovascular improvement. You have to push yourself at least a little bit. Remember the "Talk Test" from the previous chapter? You should be able to talk, but you shouldn't be able to sing. If you can belt out your favorite tune without effort, you need to pick up the pace!

Another common issue is **improper footwear**. Your old, beat-up sneakers from ten years ago aren't going to cut it. Walking puts a specific kind of stress on your feet, and you need shoes that provide good arch support and cushioning for your heels. Go to a dedicated shoe store and get fitted for a proper pair of walking or running shoes. It's a small investment that will prevent blisters, shin splints, and knee pain. Think of your shoes as the tires on your car—if they're bald and out of alignment, the whole ride is going to suffer. Take care of your feet, and they will take care of your heart.

Many people also give up because walking seems "too simple." We've been conditioned to think that if a workout isn't complicated and miserable, it isn't working. This is a dangerous myth. The best exercise is the one you will actually do. Walking is sustainable because it doesn't require a lot of prep time, it doesn't leave you feeling exhausted for the rest of the day, and it's actually enjoyable. Don't let the simplicity fool you. The benefits to your heart, your blood pressure, and your cholesterol levels are very real and very scientifically proven. Embrace the simplicity. Let it be the foundation of your success.

Finally, watch out for the **all-or-nothing trap**. If you miss a day, don't throw in the towel and decide the whole week is a wash. Just start again the next day. Life happens. Sometimes it rains, sometimes you have a late meeting, and sometimes you just don't have the energy. That's okay. The goal is to make walking a *habit*, not a perfect streak. Be kind to yourself, but stay committed to the long-term vision. Your heart is a forgiving organ; it will welcome you back to the pavement whenever you're ready.

### Reflecting on Your Journey

As we wrap up this look at the power of walking, I want you to take a moment to think about your own day there a colleague who would be open to a "walking meeting" instead of sitting in a cramped office? The opportunities are everywhere once you start looking for them. Your heart is waiting for you to make the move. It's been working for you since before you were born, and it's ready for a little help from its "second heart" in your legs.

Think about who you can invite into this journey with you. Health is contagious. When you start walking every day, people will notice. They'll see the extra spring in your step and the glow in your face. You might just inspire your spouse, your children, or your friends to start their own heart-health journey. Imagine a neighborhood where everyone is out on the sidewalks, greeting each other and taking care of their hearts together. That's the kind of world we can build, one step at a time. It starts with you, and it starts today.

Walking is truly the simplest secret to a long and vibrant life. It's the bridge between our ancient past and our healthy future. It's a way to assist your heart, clear your mind, and reclaim your vitality. You have the form, you have the science, and you have the plan. Now, all that's left is to lace up those shoes and step outside. The fresh air is waiting, the sidewalk is open, and your heart is ready to beat with a new kind of strength. I'll see you out there on the path. Let's make every step count for the rest of our lives.

**Key Takeaways for the Road Ahead**

- **Walking is a total-body heart helper.** By engaging the calf muscles, you create a "second heart" that assists in returning blood to your chest.
- **Form is everything.** Use the Power Walk technique—tall posture, vigorous arm swing, and a heel-to-toe roll—to maximize your benefits.
- **Intensity matters.** Aim for a "purposeful" pace that gets you into the target heart rate zone while still allowing you to speak.
- **Every step is a deposit.** Don't ignore incidental movement. Parking further away and taking the stairs add up to significant heart health over time.
- **Make it social.** A walking partner provides the accountability and enjoyment that make a habit stick for the long haul.

By following these principles, you are doing more than just "going for a walk." You are engaging in a sophisticated, evolutionarily designed practice that strengthens your most vital organ. You are taking ownership of your health in the simplest, most effective way possible. Your heart belongs to you, and today, you are giving it the gift of movement. Keep those feet moving, keep that head held high, and keep listening to the steady, strong rhythm of your progress. You are doing great work, and your heart knows it!

# Chapter 14
## The 90s Gym: Machines and Motivation

Imagine walking into a room filled with the rhythmic hum of spinning flywheels, the steady thud of feet hitting rubber belts, and the clanking of weight stacks. There is a specific smell to this place—a mix of ozone from the electric motors and the metallic scent of chrome. This is the modern gym, a space that has undergone a massive transformation in just a few short years. It used to be that if you wanted to find a place to sweat, you had to hunt down a basement filled with rusted iron and guys trying to look like Hercules. But things have changed. Today, the local fitness center is a bright, welcoming laboratory where you can precisely engineer your cardiovascular health using some of the most advanced technology ever developed for the human body.

The gym is no longer just for bodybuilders or elite athletes. It is a tool for every person who wants to see their pulse grow stronger and their energy levels skyrocket. When you step through those doors, you are entering a controlled environment where the variables of weather, traffic, and uneven ground are replaced by programmable resistance and digital feedback. You have a fleet of machines at your disposal, each one designed to challenge your heart in a slightly different way. Whether it is the smooth glide of a stationary bike or the relentless climb of a stair machine, you are in the driver's seat of your own physiology. This is where we take the guesswork out of fitness and replace it with a systematic approach to longevity.

I know the gym can feel a bit overwhelming if you haven't spent much time there. The flashing lights on the consoles and the sheer variety of equipment can make anyone feel like a fish out of water. But here is the thing: every single person in that room is there for the same reason you are. They want to feel better, look better, and live longer. The machines aren't there to intimidate you; they are there to serve you. They are your partners in the quest for a superior pump. By learning how to navigate this landscape of steel and cable, you are going to unlock a level of cardiovascular conditioning that just isn't possible by staying on the couch. Let's get into the specifics of how this environment actually changes the way your body works.

### The Two Types of Growth: Skeletal vs. Cardiac

When most people hear the word **hypertrophy**, they immediately think of massive biceps and broad shoulders. In the world of weightlifting, hypertrophy refers to the increase in the size of skeletal muscle cells. You lift a heavy weight, you create tiny tears in the muscle fibers, and the body repairs them by making them thicker and stronger. This is a great way to look good at the beach, but it is fundamentally different from what we are trying to achieve with our most important muscle: the heart. While both involve growth, the way the heart responds to exercise is a specialized process that determines how efficiently you can deliver oxygen to your cells.

The heart is a muscle, but it doesn't just get "big" in one way. There are actually two types of cardiac hypertrophy, and understanding the difference is key to your training strategy. The first is what we might call "athlete's heart" or **eccentric hypertrophy**. This occurs when you engage in consistent aerobic exercise, like the kind you do on a treadmill or a bike. During these activities, the heart has to pump a large volume of blood over a long period. To handle this, the chambers of the heart—specifically the left ventricle—actually stretch and expand. The muscle wall becomes more elastic, allowing the heart to fill with more blood between beats. This increases your **stroke volume**, meaning you move more blood with every single pump. This is the gold standard for cardiovascular health.

On the other hand, there is **concentric hypertrophy**, which can be caused by chronic high blood pressure or excessive, straining weightlifting without any cardio. In this case, the heart has to push against high resistance. To cope, the walls of the heart thicken and become stiff, but the chamber size stays the same or even shrinks. This makes the heart less efficient because it can't hold as much blood, and it has to work harder just to keep the circulation moving. Our goal in the gym is to promote that healthy, elastic expansion. We want a heart that is powerful because it is efficient, not because it is struggling against its own stiffness. By using the machines correctly, we are training the heart to be a high-volume pump that stays relaxed even under pressure.

This is why we focus so much on the aerobic machines in the gym. They provide the steady, rhythmic demand that encourages the heart to grow in the right way. When you spend thirty minutes on a stationary bike it how to be flexible and resilient. It is a beautiful process of adaptation. Your body sees the demand you are placing on it and says, "I need to be better at this." It then sets about remodeling your internal plumbing to make sure you have all the oxygen you need. This isn't just about burning fat; it is about rebuilding your engine from the inside out.

### The Big Three: Treadmills, Bikes, and StairMasters

If you walk into any well-equipped fitness center today, you are going to see three staples of the cardio floor. These are the workhorses of the 90s wellness movement. Each one offers a unique benefit to your heart, and knowing how to use them effectively will keep your workouts fresh and your progress steady. Let's start with the **treadmill**. This is the most versatile machine in the room. It allows you to walk or run at a perfectly consistent pace, something that is nearly impossible to do outdoors. But the real secret of the treadmill isn't the speed; it is the **incline**. By raising the deck even just a few degrees, you significantly increase the demand on your heart without having to move your legs any faster. It is a low-impact way to get your pulse into that fat-burning zone.

Next up is the **stationary bike**. This is the perfect choice for anyone who wants to protect their joints while still getting a high-intensity workout. The bike allows you to control the **resistance**, which is essentially the "weight" you are pushing with your legs. By cranking up the resistance, you force your heart to pump harder to deliver blood to those large leg muscles. Many modern bikes also come with pre-programmed "hill" or "interval" routines. These are fantastic because they take the decision-making out of your hands. The machine will automatically change the difficulty, forcing your heart to adapt to different levels of stress throughout the session. It is like having a personal trainer built right into the console.

Then we have the legendary **StairMaster**. This machine became a sensation for a reason—it is perhaps the most effective tool for building cardiovascular endurance and lower-body strength simultaneously. Climbing stairs is a vertical challenge, meaning you are fighting gravity with every single step. This puts a massive demand on the heart. However, there is a common mistake people make on this machine: they lean on the handrails. If you are supporting your weight with your arms, you are cheating your heart out of the work it needs. To get the full benefit, you must stand upright and let your legs do the heavy lifting. Your heart rate will soar, and your calves and glutes will feel the burn, but that is exactly where the transformation happens.

When using these machines, I want you to focus on the **Quick Start** button. Most beginners get bogged down trying to enter their age, weight, and favorite color into the computer before they even start moving. Forget all that for now. Just get on the machine, hit Quick Start, and begin at a low level. As you feel the technology. The goal is to get your heart rate up, not to become a computer programmer. Once you are comfortable with the basics, you beat of your heart.

### From Dungeons to Wellness Centers

It is fascinating to look at how far the gym has come. If we go back twenty or thirty years, the "gym" was a very different place. It was often located in a dark, poorly ventilated basement. The equipment was made of heavy, clanking iron, and the atmosphere was one of pure, raw strength. These were the "bodybuilding dungeons" where men went to lift massive weights and grunt through their sets. There was very little focus on heart health, and you certainly wouldn't find many women or seniors in those spaces. It was an intimidating environment that prioritized the size of the muscle over the health of the individual. Cardiovascular exercise was often seen as an afterthought, something you did only if you were trying to "cut" for a competition People began to realize that looking strong wasn't the same as being healthy. The medical community started shouting from the rooftops about the importance of aerobic capacity and cholesterol management. In response, gyms began to evolve. They moved out of the basements and into bright, airy retail spaces. They traded the rusted iron for sleek, chrome-plated machines and high-tech electronics. This was the birth of the "wellness center." These new clubs were designed to be inclusive, welcoming people of all ages and fitness levels. The focus shifted from "how much can you bench?" to "how healthy is your heart?"

This transition was fueled by the realization that the heart is the foundation of all physical performance. You could have the biggest muscles in the world, but if your heart couldn't deliver oxygen to them, they were useless. The introduction of computerized cardio equipment changed everything. Suddenly data empowered people to take control of their health in a way that was never before possible. The gym became a place of education and empowerment, a place where you could learn the science of your own body while you worked to improve it.

Today, when you walk into a modern gym, you are standing on the shoulders of this evolution. You have access to tools that would have seemed like science fiction to the gym-goers of the 1970s. You have clean facilities, expert staff, and a community of people who are all working toward a common goal. This environment is designed to help you succeed. It removes the machine that it is.

## The Power of Resistance Settings

Many people make the mistake of thinking that "resistance" is only for building muscle. They see the dial on the bike or the level setting on the treadmill and they think, "I don't want to get bulky legs, so I'll just keep it easy." Let me tell you, that is a major misconception. Resistance is one of the most powerful tools you have for strengthening your heart. When you increase the resistance on a cardio machine, you aren't just making the workout "harder" for your legs; you are increasing the **peripheral resistance** that your heart has to pump against. This is a form of strength training for your cardiac muscle.

Think of it this way: when you are on a bike with no resistance, your legs are moving fast but they aren't doing much work. Your heart rate might go up because of the speed, but the heart isn't really being challenged to push. Now, imagine you turn that dial up. Suddenly, every stroke of the pedal requires effort. Your leg muscles contract with more force, which squeezes the blood vessels and makes it harder for the heart to move blood through them. To overcome this, the heart has to contract more powerfully. This strengthens the walls of the heart and improves its ability to handle pressure. It is like the difference between a car cruising on a flat road and a car pulling a trailer up a hill. you in your target heart rate zone. You don't want so much resistance that you can only move the pedals by jumping steadily, and you can feel your muscles working, but you can still maintain a consistent pace for twenty or thirty minutes. This balance of speed and resistance is the secret to maximum cardiac efficiency. It forces the heart to adapt to both volume and pressure, giving you the best of both worlds.

I recommend playing with these settings during your workout. Don't just set it and forget it. Try a "pyramid" approach: start with low resistance for five minutes to keeps your heart on its toes. It prevents your body from becoming too efficient at a single level of effort, which is how you avoid those frustrating fitness plateaus. Your heart is an incredibly adaptable organ, but it needs a reason to change. By varied resistance, you are giving it a new challenge every single day, ensuring that you continue to see improvements in your endurance and your overall health.

### Interval Training on Machines

If you want to see the fastest possible results in your cardiovascular fitness, you need to incorporate **interval training** into your gym routine. We touched on this with walking, but the gym machines take this concept to a whole new level. Because you can precisely control the intensity work and periods of lower-intensity recovery. This "on-off" pattern is like a miracle drug for your heart. It pushes your aerobic capacity higher than steady-state exercise ever could, and it does it in a fraction of the time.

Here is why it works so well. During the high-intensity burst, you are pushing your heart to its limit. You are demanding that it pump as much blood as possible to keep up with the oxygen needs of your muscles. This creates a powerful stimulus for growth and adaptation. Then, during the recovery period, you aren't stopping; you are just slowing down. faster your heart rate drops after a hard effort, the more fit you are. By practicing this repeatedly, you are training your nervous system to be more efficient at regulating your pulse.

You can do intervals on any machine. On a treadmill, you might alternate between two minutes of walking on a flat surface and one minute of walking at a steep incline. On a stationary bike, you might do thirty seconds of "sprinting" at a high resistance followed by ninety seconds of easy pedaling. The possibilities are endless. The beauty of the gym is that the machine keeps track of the time and the intensity for you. You don't have to worry about looking at your watch or finding a hill; you just focus on the effort. It is a highly efficient way to spend your time. You can get more heart-health benefits from twenty minutes of intervals than you can from forty-five minutes of steady, easy movement.

However, I want to give you a word of caution. Interval training is intense. You should only start incorporating these high-effort bursts after you have built a solid foundation of at least a few weeks of steady-state exercise. Listen to your body. During the "on" periods, you should feel like you are working hard—you should be huffing and puffing—but you should never feel pain or dizziness. If you ever feel like your heart is skipping a beat or you feel lightheaded, stop immediately and rest. We are looking for a challenge, not a crisis. Start with one interval session a week and gradually increase as your heart becomes more resilient. This is the fast track to a powerful, efficient pump.

### Gym Etiquette for Beginners

Before you head out to your local club, let's talk about the unwritten rules of the gym. Every social environment has its own set of "etiquette" guidelines, and the gym is no different. Knowing these rules will help you feel more confident and ensure that everyone has a positive experience. First and foremost: is a good thing! But nobody wants to use a machine that is covered in someone else's moisture. Most gyms provide spray bottles and paper towels; make it a habit to wipe down every surface you touch as soon as you are finished. It is a simple gesture of respect for your fellow members.

Second, be mindful of **time limits** on the machines. During busy hours, most gyms have a thirty-minute limit on popular equipment like treadmills and StairMasters. Even if there isn't a sign, if you see people waiting, don't hog the machine for an hour. If you need a longer workout, consider splitting your time between two different machines. This actually benefits your heart by providing more variety, and it keeps the flow of the gym moving smoothly. Along those same lines, try not to "camp out" on a machine while you are resting or checking your pulse. If you aren't actively using the equipment, step aside so someone else can. The gym is a community space, and it works best when everyone is considerate of each other's time.

Third, let's talk about **safety**. This is the most important part of gym etiquette. Before you start a machine, make sure you know how to stop it. Every treadmill has a big red "Emergency Stop" button or a clip that attaches to your clothing. Use it! If you trip or feel unwell, you need to be able to kill the power instantly. Also, never step onto a moving treadmill belt. Wait for it to come to a complete stop before you get on or off. When using weight machines or resistance settings, make sure the pins are fully inserted and everything is secure. If you aren't sure how a machine works, **ask the staff**. That is what they are there for. There is no shame in asking for a demonstration; in fact, the staff would much rather show you the right way than have to fill out an accident report.

Finally, remember that the gym is a "no-judgment zone." It is easy to look around and feel like everyone else knows what they are doing while you are just fumbling through. But the truth is, most people are so focused on their own workout that they aren't even looking at you. And the people who *are* looking are usually thinking, "Good for them for being here." We are all on the same team. Whether you are walking at two miles per hour or running at ten, you are doing something incredible for your heart. Hold your head high, follow the rules, and focus on your own progress. You belong in that room just as much as anyone else.

### Variation: The Key to Long-Term Success

One of the biggest pitfalls in any fitness routine is **boredom**. If you do the exact same thirty-minute walk on the exact same treadmill every single day, eventually your mind is going to check out. And more importantly, your body is going to adapt. Our bodies are remarkably efficient at finding the easiest way to do a task. Once your heart gets used to a specific routine, it stops needing to change. This is what we call a plateau. To keep your heart growing stronger and your motivation high, you must introduce variation into your gym life. The gym is perfect for this because of the sheer variety of tools at your disposal.

I want you to think of your gym time as a rotation. Maybe on Monday, you use the treadmill for an incline walk. On Wednesday, you hit the stationary bike for some high-resistance intervals. On Friday, you tackle the StairMaster for a steady climb. This "cross-training" approach ensures that you are challenging your cardiovascular system from multiple angles. The treadmill works your heart through speed and incline; the bike works it through resistance and leg speed; the stair climber works it through vertical power. Each machine stresses the heart in a slightly different way, leading to a more well-rounded and resilient cardiovascular system.

Variation also helps prevent overuse injuries. If to the bike or the elliptical, you give those joints a break while still giving your heart the workout it needs. This longevity is crucial. We aren't just training for next week; we are training for the next thirty years. By keeping things fresh, you make it much more likely that you will stick with the habit for the long haul. You will find yourself looking forward to the different challenges of each machine, rather than dreading the "same old" routine.

Don't be afraid to try something new. Most gyms have machines you might have never seen before, like rowing machines or "upper body" ergometers. Each one of these is an opportunity to learn more about your body and give your heart a new stimulus. If you feel like your progress has stalled, or if you find yourself making excuses to skip the gym, that is a clear sign that you need to change things up. Throw a curveball at your physiology. Try a new machine, change your interval timing, or even just work out at a different time of day. Keep your heart guessing, and it will keep rewarding you with better health and more energy.

### Overcoming Gym Intimidation

Let's be honest: for a lot of people, the hardest part of the gym isn't the workout—it's just walking through the front door. We've all had those thoughts: "I'm too out of shape to be here," or “Everyone is going to stare at me.” This is what we call gym intimidation, and it is a very real barrier for many people. But I want to give you a different perspective. Think of the gym as a **tool**, like a hammer or a screwdriver. You wouldn’t feel intimidated by a screwdriver, would you? It is just an object designed to help you do a job. The treadmill is no different. It is a piece of steel and plastic designed to help you strengthen your heart. It doesn’t have an opinion of you.

Most of the people you see in the gym who look like they “live there” actually have a lot of respect for beginners. They know how hard it is to start. They remember their own first day when they felt lost and out of place. The fitness community is generally one of the most supportive groups you’ll ever find. We are all united by the struggle against gravity and the desire for a better life. When you see someone who is very fit, don’t look at them as a source of shame; look at them as a source of **information**. Notice their form, their intensity, and their consistency. They are living proof that the system works.

One great way to beat intimidation is to have a plan. Don’t just wander around aimlessly looking at the machines. Before you even leave your house, decide exactly what you are going to do. “Today, I am going to do twenty minutes on the bike at level five.” When you have a mission, you feel more purposeful. You walk in, go straight to your machine, and get to work. This focus helps block out the “noise” of the room and keeps your anxiety at bay. You aren’t there to win a beauty pageant or a strength competition; you are there to do a specific job for your heart. Once you get into the rhythm of the machine, everything else tends to fade away.

Finally, remember that everyone starts somewhere. Even the most elite athlete had a first day. The only difference between you and the person who has been coming for ten years is time and consistency. You have the same potential to transform your health that they do. Every time you show up, you are building confidence. After a few weeks, the "newness" will wear off, and the gym will start to feel like a second home. You'll have your favorite treadmill, you'll know the staff by name, and you'll feel a sense of ownership over your health. The intimidation will be replaced by a sense of pride. You are taking charge of your life, and that is something to be celebrated.

**Your Action Plan: Into the Chrome**

It is time to turn this information into action. I want you to make a commitment to yourself to explore the world of gym-based cardio this week. This isn't about running a marathon on your first day; it is about familiarizing yourself with the environment and the tools at your disposal. Follow these three steps to get started on your gym journey.

1. **Visit a local gym and take a tour.** Don't even worry about working out the first time. Just walk in, ask for a tour, and look around. Check out the cardio area, see where the towels and water fountains are, and get a feel for the atmosphere. Most gyms will even give you a free day pass to try things out. This "scouting mission" removes the mystery and makes your first actual workout much less stressful.

2. **Try the stationary bike for 15 minutes at a moderate resistance.** Once you are ready for your first session, the bike is the perfect entry point. It is easy to use, it is low-impact, and you can clearly see how the resistance settings affect your effort. Aim for a pace that

feels like a brisk walk. You should be able to feel your heart beating faster, but you shouldn't be gasping for air. This short session is just to get your feet wet and prove to yourself that you can do it.

3. **Learn how to use the 'Quick Start' button on a treadmill.** On your next visit, step onto the treadmill. Don't worry about the programs or the incline yet. Just find that big green Quick Start button and get the belt moving at a slow walk. Practice increasing and decreasing the speed. Get comfortable with the safety features. Once you feel confident, try walking for ten minutes at a pace that makes you feel "purposeful."

As you complete these steps, pay attention to how your body responds. Notice the feeling of your blood circulating more vigorously. Notice the sense of accomplishment as you master a new piece of equipment. You are no longer just "thinking" about your heart health; you are actively engineering it. You are using the best technology available to give your heart the workout it deserves. This is the beginning of a new chapter in your fitness story, one where you have all the tools you need to succeed. I'll be right there with you as you continue to explore the incredible potential of your own human pump.

### Common Mistakes to Avoid

To get the most out of your gym time, we need to address a few common habits that can stall your progress or even lead to injury. One of the biggest mistakes I see on the **StairMaster** is people using the side rails to support their body weight. If your arms are doing the work, your heart and legs are not. This drastically reduces the caloric burn and the cardiovascular stimulus. If you can't maintain the pace without leaning on the rails, simply slow the machine down. It is much better to go yet, let your arms swing naturally as if you were climbing real stairs.

Another frequent error is **not knowing how to stop the machine** in an emergency. This is particularly true for treadmills. Before you even hit start, locate the stop button. If the machine has a safety clip, use it! It attaches to your waistband and will instantly kill the power if you move too far back on the belt. I've seen too many people try to jump off a moving treadmill because they couldn't find the button, which is a recipe for a twisted ankle or worse. Safety is the foundation of consistency. If you feel safe, you are much more likely to push yourself and come back for your next session.

Finally, avoid the trap of **sticking to only one machine forever**. I see people who have been using the same elliptical for three years at the same intensity. While any movement is better than none, this lack of variety leads to stagnation. Your heart is an expert at adapting. If you give it the same challenge every day walk, try the bike. If you always use the "Hill" program, try "Random" or "Intervals." This constant novelty is what keeps the heart growing and the metabolism humming. Don't be a creature of habit; be a creature of growth.

By avoiding these pitfalls, you are making your gym time twice as effective. smarter, not just harder. Remember, the goal isn't just to "do the time" on the machine; the goal is to create a specific physiological response in your heart. By using proper form, prioritizing safety, and embracing variety, you are giving sophisticated approach to training.

## Reflecting on Your Environment

Take a look at your current relationship with the idea of "the gym." Does it feel like a place of judgment, or a place of opportunity of the past. In our modern understanding of health, the gym is simply a tool—a high-tech laboratory where you can precisely measure and improve your most vital organ. It is a space designed to support your goals, regardless of where you are starting from today.

Think about how you can view the gym as a partner in your health. Instead of seeing it as a chore, try to see it as a gift you give to your heart. It is a place where you can step away from the stresses of daily life and focus entirely on your own well-being. The hum of the machines and the steady rhythm of your movement can be incredibly meditative. It is a time for you to connect with your body and listen to what it needs. Your heart has been working for you every second of every day since before purpose?

You have the knowledge, you have the technology, and you have the plan. The only thing left is to step through those doors and get started. The world of chrome and cables is waiting for you, and every climb on the stairs is a victory. Keep moving, keep pushing, and keep listening to the strong, steady beat of your own progress. You are well on your way to a lifetime of heart-healthy living, and the gym is the perfect place to make it happen.

# Chapter 15
## *Flexibility and the Fluid Heart*

Have you ever noticed how a stiff rubber band behaves compared to a fresh, supple one? If you try to stretch that old, dried-out piece of elastic, it resists, cracks, and eventually snaps. But a new one? It gives, it flows, and it returns to its original shape without a hitch. Your body operates on the exact same principle. We spend so much time talking about the "pump" and the "burn" that we often forget about the "flow." If your muscles are locked up like a rusty gate, your cardiovascular system has to fight an uphill battle every single second of the day. Flexibility isn't just for gymnasts or people who want to touch their toes at the beach; it is a fundamental requirement for a heart that wants to beat with ease and efficiency.

In this chapter, we are moving away from the high-intensity clatter of the weight room and the steady drone of the treadmill to focus on the quiet, essential art of lengthening. We often think of our health as a series of aggressive actions—running faster, lifting heavier, eating stricter. But sometimes, the most profound thing you can do for your longevity isn't just becoming more limber. You are literally opening up the pipes of your circulatory system. A fluid body creates The Mechanical Connection: Why Tightness Stops the Pump

To understand why flexibility matters for your pulse, we need to look at the plumbing. Your blood vessels don't just float in a vacuum; they are woven through and around your muscles and connective tissues. When a muscle is chronically tight—perhaps because you sit at a desk all day or because you've been pushing hard on the StairMaster without cooling down—it becomes dense and hard. This physical hardness creates a form of external pressure on your arteries and veins. It's like trying to run water through a garden hose that has a heavy rock sitting on top of it. The pump has to push with significantly more force just to move the same amount of fluid.

This is what medical professionals call peripheral resistance. When your limbs are tight, your heart must increase the blood pressure to shove oxygenated blood into those constricted areas. If this happens for an hour, it's no" off the hose. You are creating a path of least resistance for your blood, which allows your resting heart rate to drop and your blood pressure to stabilize. It is the ultimate form of internal maintenance.

Furthermore, flexibility impacts ribcage and diaphragm. If your chest muscles are tight and your shoulders are hunched forward, your lungs cannot fully expand. This leads to shallow, rapid breathing, which signals the nervous system to stay in a state of "fight or flight." This elevated stress state keeps your heart rate high and your arteries constricted. Stretching the "heart-opening" areas—the pectorals and the thoracic spine—allows for deeper, more efficient breaths. This means more oxygen per inhalation, which translates to less work for your cardiac we navigate the 1990s, we are seeing a massive shift in how the average person views fitness. For decades, the Western model was entirely about "no pain, no gain." If you weren't sweating or straining, it like Yoga and Tai Chi, which were once relegated to the fringes of society, are now becoming staples in neighborhood health clubs. People are realizing that the ancient sages were onto something: you cannot have true strength without suppleness.

Now, we understand it as a discipline in its own right. The introduction of these "mind-body" practices has taught us that the heart isn't just a mechanical pump; it's an organ that responds to the state of our nervous system. When we hold a deep stretch and focus on our breath, we are engaging the parasympathetic nervous system—the "rest and digest" mode. This is the only time the heart truly gets to recover and repair itself. By embracing these older traditions, we are giving our modern bodies a chance to find balance in a world that never seems to slow down.

### The Heart-Opening Routine: Your Daily Reset

I want to introduce you to a specific set of movements designed to counteract the "closed-off" posture that most of us adopt throughout the day. Think about your typical afternoon: you're likely leaning over a steering wheel, a keyboard, or a dinner plate. This position collapses the chest, rounds the shoulders, and tightens the hips. It is the physical embodiment of stress. The following routine is designed to reverse this trend and open up the "housing" of your heart. These aren't just stretches; they are postural corrections that facilitate better blood flow and lung capacity.

- **The Doorway Chest Stretch:** Stand in a doorway and place your forearms on the doorframe with your elbows at shoulder height. Slowly lean forward until you feel a gentle pull across your chest and the without restriction.

- **The Kneeling Hip Flexor Stretch:** Kneel on one knee with the other foot flat in front of you. Shift your weight forward slightly, keeping your torso upright. Most people have incredibly tight hips from sitting, which actually pulls on the lower back and affects overall circulation to the lower extremities. Opening the hips helps the blood return to the heart more easily.

- **The Cat-Cow Flow:** On your hands and knees, alternate between arching your back and looking up (Cow) and rounding your spine while tucking your chin (Cat). This moves the spine through its full range of motion and helps massage the internal organs, including the area surrounding the heart.

- **The Seated Spinal Twist:** Sit on the floor with your legs extended. Cross one foot over the opposite knee and gently twist your torso toward the upright knee. This rotation helps "wring out" the tension in the mid-back, which is where many of us store the physical manifestations of emotional stress.

The key to this routine is **breath-movement coordination**. You should never be gasping or holding your breath while you stretch. Instead, try to time your movements so that you are expanding as you inhale and sinking deeper into the stretch as you exhale. This rhythm creates a sedative effect on the heart. It tells your brain that you are safe, which allows your blood vessels to dilate and your pulse to find a calm, steady cadence. If you find yourself gritting your teeth, you've gone too far. Back off and find the "sweet spot" where the muscle is lengthening but the body remains relaxed.

### The Perils of 'Ballistic' Stretching

Before you get started, we need to clear up a very common mistake that has persisted since the old gym days: bouncing. You've probably seen people at the track bouncing up and down while trying to touch their toes. This is called ballistic stretching, and for the average person looking for heart health, it is a terrible idea. When you bounce, you trigger something called the "stretch reflex." Your muscles sense a sudden change in length and, fearing a tear, they actually contract to protect themselves. You end up fighting your own body, which increases tension rather than releasing it.

For our purposes, we use **static stretching**. This means you move into the position slowly and hold it. No movement, no jerking, just a steady, calm presence in the stretch. This spikes in blood pressure that can occur with jerky, high-effort movements. Remember, we are trying to teach the heart how to be quiet and fluid. Bouncing is the language of aggression; holding is the language of recovery. Stick to the slow road, and your arteries will thank you for the smooth ride.

### The Evening Stretch: A Bridge to Better Sleep

Timing is everything. While a quick warm-up stretch before exercise is fine, the real, restorative sleep your heart needs. During the day, your body is bombarded by adrenaline and cortisol—the stress hormones. These chemicals keep your heart rate elevated and your muscles on edge

By dedicating just ten minutes before bed to a full-body stretch, you are performing a manual override on your nervous system. As you lengthen your muscles, you are sending a signal to your brain to stop the production of stress hormones and start the production of melatonin and other recovery agents. This "downshifting" is vital for cardiac health. A heart that can quickly transition from the demands of the day to a state of deep rest is a resilient heart. It's the difference between a car that you turn off and let cool down versus one that you leave idling in the garage all night. Don't let your "engine" idle; use flexibility to shut it down properly.

1. **Create a Quiet Environment:** Turn down the lights and turn off the television. This isn't just about the muscles; it's about the senses. A and back. These areas hold the most tension and require the most blood flow. When they relax, the systemic effect is massive.

2. **Hold for 30 Seconds:** It takes time for the nervous system to give the "all clear" to a tight muscle. Research suggests that thirty seconds is the minimum time required to achieve a lasting change in muscle length.

3. **Practice Nasal Breathing:** Breathe only through your nose during your routine. This naturally slows the breath and keeps the heart in a rhythmic, aerobic state.

If you make this a habit, you will likely find that you wake up feeling less "heavy." That morning stiffness we often attribute to age is frequently just the leftover tension from the day before. By clearing the slate every night, you start each morning with a body that is ready to move and a heart that isn't already tired from fighting its own housing. It is a simple, free, and incredibly effective way to add years to your life and life to your years.

## Flexibility as a Life Philosophy

There is a deeper lesson here that goes beyond the physical fibers of your calves or your chest. To have a healthy heart, you must also cultivate a flexible mind. We live in a world that demands we be rigid—rigid in our schedules, rigid in our opinions, and rigid in our expectations. This mental rigidity creates a physical "armoring" in the body. When we are stressed or defensive, we physically tighten our core and shorten our breath. Over time, this becomes our default setting, and our heart pays the price.

Learning to be flexible in your body teaches you how to be flexible in your life. When you encounter a "stretch" in your daily routine—a stressful meeting, a traffic jam, a difficult conversation—you can lean into it rather than snapping. You learn to breathe through the discomfort and wait for the release. This emotional resilience is just as important for preventing heart disease as any diet or exercise routine. A heart that can "bend" with the winds of fortune is a heart that will not break. As you work on your physical suppleness, take a moment to consider where you might be holding unnecessary rigidity in your thoughts. Let those go, too. Your pulse will feel the difference.

## Common Mistakes and How to Fix Them

Even with the best intentions, it's easy to fall into habits that undermine your progress. The most common pitfall is **holding the breath**. When we feel a bit of discomfort in a stretch, our natural instinct is to gasp or hold our air. This is the exact opposite of what we want! Holding your breath increases internal thoracic pressure, which actually puts more strain on the heart. If you can't breathe comfortably, you are stretching too hard. The breath is your gauge; if it's smooth, you're doing great. If it's jagged, back off.

Another mistake is **pushing to the point of pain**. We've been conditioned to think that "more is better," but in flexibility training, "enough is perfect." You are looking for a sensation of "comfortable tension." It should feel like a deep, satisfying pull, almost like a yawn for your muscles. If you feel sharp, stabbing, or electric sensations, stop immediately. You are likely pulling on a nerve or a tendon rather than lengthening the muscle belly. Respect your boundaries. Your heart doesn't need you to be a contortionist; it just needs you to be open.

Lastly, don't ignore **symmetry**. Most of us have one side that is tighter than the other—usually due to how we carry a bag, sit in a car, or even which leg we lead with when we walk. If you only stretch your "good" side, you create imbalances that can lead to skewed posture and inefficient movement. Always spend an equal amount of time on both sides, and perhaps even an extra thirty seconds on the tighter side. A balanced body allows the heart to sit centered and move blood evenly to both halves of the "machine."

### Your Action Plan: The Fluid Heart

It is time to put these principles into practice. Flexibility isn't a destination; it's a daily maintenance requirement. You don't "get flexible" and then stop; you move to stay fluid. I want you to commit to these three simple steps starting tonight. Don't wait for Monday or for a new gym membership. You have everything you need right where you are.

1. **Perform a 10-minute full-body stretch before bed.** Focus on the big areas: the hamstrings, the hips nightly gift to your cardiovascular system.

2. **Focus on deep, slow breaths during each stretch.** Use your breath to "melt" the tension. Imagine your breath traveling to the tightest part of your body and carrying the stress away as you exhale. This mental focus doubles the effectiveness of the physical movement.

3. **Hold each stretch for at least 30 seconds—no bouncing!** Use a clock or simply count thirty slow, deep heartbeats. This ensures that you are actually changing the tissue rather than just temporarily pulling on it. Stay still, stay calm, and let the muscle release on its own time.

As you move through these steps, pay close attention to the sensation of your body "opening up." You might feel a slight tingling or a sense of warmth in your limbs; that is the sound of your blood finally reaching the places it has been struggling to go. It is a feeling of relief. Your heart is no longer struggling against a suit of armor. It is beating in a body that is spacious, resilient, and ready for anything.

Think about where you hold the most tension. Is it in your jaw? Your shoulders? Your lower back? How does that tension feel when you try to take a deep, full breath? Usually, you'll find that the tension acts like a cage, restricting the very air you need to live. By identifying these "hot spots," you can target them with your new routine. Over the next week, notice how your overall energy levels change. When your heart doesn't have to fight your muscles, you'll find you have a lot more "fuel in the tank" for the things you actually enjoy doing. You're not just becoming more flexible; you're becoming more alive. Keep flowing, keep breathing, and remember that a supple body is the best home a heart could ever have.

# Chapter 16
## Recovery:
## The Heart's Quiet Time

Ever feel like you're running on empty, even when you've been hitting the gym every single morning? Maybe you're following the low-fat diet to the letter, and you're crushing those aerobic sessions on the stationary bike, but you still feel sluggish when you wake up. Well, friend, there is a very good reason for that. We often get caught up in the "more is better" trap. We think that if thirty minutes of exercise is good, then sixty minutes must be twice as good. But let's set the record straight: your body doesn't actually get stronger while you're lifting those weights or pounding the pavement. That is just the stimulus. The actual growth, the real improvement, and the vital repair of your cardiac system happen when you stop. That is right. Your heart gets better when you are doing absolutely nothing.

Think about the rhythm of life itself. Everything has a pulse—an expansion and a contraction, a rise and a fall. Your heart follows this same beat. It spends half its life in systole, contracting to push blood out, and the other half in diastole, relaxing to let the blood back in. If you never let the "relaxation" phase of your lifestyle take place, you are essentially asking your body to live in a permanent state of contraction. That is a recipe for burnout, injury, and a heart that wears out long before its time. Recovery isn't a sign of weakness or a lack of dedication. It is a strategic, physiological requirement for anyone who wants to live a long, vibrant life. Without rest, the work you do is just a slow way of tearing yourself down.

## The Anatomy of Repair: How Your Heart Heals

When we talk about fitness, we usually focus on the "tearing down" phase. When you engage in a vigorous aerobic workout, you are putting stress on your cardiac muscle fibers. You are making your heart beat faster, pushing more blood through the chambers, and stretching the walls of your arteries. This is good stress, but it is stress nonetheless. To adapt to this demand and become more efficient, your body needs a period of downtime to conduct what we call the remodeling phase. This is a complex biological process where your cells go to work like a construction crew at night, fixing the wear and tear and reinforcing the structure so it can handle more load tomorrow.

During deep sleep and dedicated rest periods, your body enters an anabolic state. This is the opposite of the catabolic state you are in during exercise. In an anabolic state, your system releases growth hormones and repairs damaged tissues. For this phase, those tiny bits of wear and tear don't get fixed. They accumulate. Over time, this leads to chronic fatigue and a decrease in your "ejection fraction," which is just a fancy way of saying how much blood your heart can pump with each beat. By resting, you are literally giving your heart the materials and the time it needs to rebuild itself into a high-performance engine.

There is also the matter of the nervous system. Your heart is controlled by the autonomic nervous system, which has two branches: the sympathetic (the "gas pedal") and the parasympathetic (the "brake"). High-intensity exercise and the stresses of daily life keep that gas pedal floored. If you don't intentionally engage the brake through recovery and sleep, your heart rate stays slightly elevated even when you think you're relaxed. This constant "revving" of the engine wastes energy and puts unnecessary strain on your valves. True recovery allows the parasympathetic system to take the wheel, lowering your resting heart rate and allowing your cardiovascular system to operate at a much lower, more efficient pressure. It's like taking your car in for an oil change and a tune-up rather than just driving it until the smoke starts pouring out from under the hood.

### Rest through the Ages: From the 'Rest Cure' to Now

Our understanding of rest has changed dramatically over the last century. If you lived in the late 1800s, doctors were obsessed with something called "neurasthenia," which they described as a total depletion of the body's nervous energy. The solution back then was the "Rest Cure." Invented by Dr. Silas Weir Mitchell, this treatment involved weeks or even months of total bed rest. Patients weren't allowed to read, write, or even feed themselves. The idea was that the body was like a battery that had run dry, and the only way to recharge it was absolute stillness. While this might sound like a dream vacation to a busy person today, it was actually quite extreme and often led to muscle atrophy and depression. They had the right idea about the importance of rest, but they didn't understand the balance.

As we moved into the mid began to be seen as laziness. In the 1970s and 80s, the fitness boom pushed the idea that you should be "going for the gold" every single day. We were told that if we weren't sweating, we weren't improving. But as we've landed here in the 1990s, we've finally found the middle ground.

We now know that the 19th-century doctors were right about the need for recovery, but the modern science tells us that recovery doesn't have to mean lying in a dark room for a month. We now distinguish between **passive recovery** (like sleep) and **active recovery** (like a gentle walk).

Active recovery is a concept that would have baffled people a hundred years ago. It's the idea that doing a very light, low-intensity activity can actually help you recover faster than doing nothing at all. When you take a slow walk on your "off" day, you're keeping the blood moving through your muscles without putting any real stress on your heart. This gentle circulation helps flush out metabolic waste products and delivers fresh nutrients to the tissues that are trying to heal. It's the perfect marriage of the ancient wisdom of rest and the modern science of movement. We've learned that the heart doesn't want to be stagnant, but it also doesn't want to be whipped like a horse every single day. It wants a rhythm that includes both the effort of the climb and the peace of the summit.

### The 90s Sleep Hygiene Checklist

Now, let's talk about the most powerful recovery tool in your arsenal: sleep. You can buy all the fancy vitamins and expensive sneakers you want, but if you aren't getting high-quality shut-eye, your heart health is going to suffer. During the night, your heart rate and blood pressure naturally drop to their lowest levels. This gives your arteries a much-needed break from the constant pressure of daily life. To make sure you're getting the most out of these hours, we need to look at your sleep hygiene. This isn't about how often you wash your sheets; it's about creating an environment that signals to your heart that it is safe to power down.

- **The Darkness Factor:** Your body is hardwired to respond to light. Even a small amount of light from a digital clock or a streetlamp can interfere with the production of melatonin, the hormone that helps you stay in deep sleep. Use heavy curtains or a sleep mask to make your room as dark as a cave.

- **Cool it Down:** Your body temperature needs to drop slightly for you to enter the most restorative stages of sleep. A room that is too warm will keep your heart rate higher than it should be. Keep your thermostat set between 65 and 68 degrees Fahrenheit for the best results.

- **Ditch the Caffeine Early:** That afternoon cup of coffee might seem harmless, but caffeine has a half-life of about six hours. If you have a cup at 4:00 PM, half of it is still in your system at 10:00 PM, keeping your heart "awake" even if your eyes are closed. Try to cut off the caffeine by noon.

- **The Alcohol Myth:** Many people think a nightcap helps them sleep. While it might help you fall asleep faster, alcohol actually disrupts your sleep cycles and prevents you from entering deep REM sleep. It also causes your heart rate to stay elevated throughout the night as your liver works to process the toxins.

- **Silence the Noise:** If you live in a noisy neighborhood, use a white noise machine or a fan. Sudden sounds can trigger a "startle response" that spikes your heart rate and pulls you out of deep recovery mode, even if you don't fully wake up.

When you follow this checklist, you aren't just "sleeping." You are conducting a nightly maintenance session on your cardiovascular system. If you wake up feeling refreshed and alert without needing three cups of coffee to function, you know your heart has had a successful recovery period. If you're waking up groggy and "heavy," it's time to look at your environment and see where the "leaks" in your recovery are happening. Remember, the quality of your sleep determines the quality of your next workout.

### Overtraining: The Heart

This happens when the volume and intensity of your exercise exceed your body's ability to recover. It's a state of chronic stress that can actually damage the very heart you are trying to protect. When you overtrain, your body is in a constant state of "fight or flight." Your cortisol levels skyrocket, your immune system weakens, and your heart becomes irritable. You might start experiencing palpitations, or you might find that your resting heart rate is ten beats higher than it usually is. These are not signs of "working hard"; they are your heart's way of screaming for a break.

One of the biggest mistakes people make is trying to "push through" extreme fatigue. They think that if they just have more willpower, they can overcome the exhaustion. But your heart doesn't care about your willpower; it cares about its cellular energy stores. When you are overtrained, your heart's ability to respond to exercise diminishes. You'll find that you can't get your heart rate up into your target zone, or that it takes forever for your pulse to return to normal after a set. This is a sign of cardiac fatigue. If you see these signs, the best thing you can do for your fitness is to stop exercising for a few days. It feels counterintuitive, but those few days of rest will do more for your performance than another week of grinding through the pain.

Another common mistake is the "weekend warrior" mentality—trying to "catch up" on sleep or exercise during the two days you have off from work. Your heart thrives on consistency, not extremes. You can't make up for five nights of five-hour sleep by sleeping for twelve hours on Sunday. All that does is throw off your body's internal clock, a phenomenon we call "social jet lag." Instead, aim for a steady rhythm. It is much better to do thirty minutes of exercise five days a week with two rest days than it is to do three hours of exercise on Saturday and Sunday and nothing during the week. Consistency is the language of the heart; intensity is just the punctuation.

### Your Recovery Action Plan

It's time to move from theory into practice. We are going to build a recovery routine that is just as structured and disciplined as your exercise routine. Most people fail at recovery because they treat it as an afterthought. They think, "I'll rest if I have time." But you will never "have time" unless you make it. You need to schedule your rest with the same priority you give to a business meeting or a doctor's appointment. Here is your three-step plan to ensure your heart gets the quiet time it deserves.

1. **The 30-Minute Shift:** Starting tonight, I want you to go to bed 30 minutes earlier than you usually do. Don't use that time to read or watch the news. Just get into bed and let your body settle. This extra half hour of rest can

add up to three and a half hours of additional recovery per week. That is a massive boost to your cardiac repair cycle. Most of us are chronically sleep-deprived, and this small shift is the easiest way to start closing that gap.

2. **The Digital Sunset:** An hour before your head hits the pillow, turn off the television and put away any bright screens. The blue light emitted by modern electronics tricks your brain into thinking it's daytime, which keeps your heart rate elevated and suppresses sleep hormones. Instead, try listening to some calm music, stretching gently (as we discussed in the last chapter), or engaging in a relaxing hobby. This creates a "buffer zone" between the stress of the day and the rest of the night.

3. **The Mandatory Rest Day:** Choose one day every week where you do absolutely no strenuous exercise. No "quick runs," no "light lifting"—just rest. If you feel like you must move, go for a leisurely walk through the park or spend some time playing with your kids. This full day of rest allows your central nervous system to reset and your glycogen stores to replenish. It's the day when your heart does its most profound remodeling. If you're worried about losing progress, don't be. You'll find that you come back the next day stronger, faster, and more motivated than if you had pushed through.

By implementing these three steps, you are taking a proactive stance on your health. You are recognizing that you are a biological organism, not a machine. Even the most powerful engines need to be turned off and cooled down. When you give your heart this quiet time, you are investing in its longevity. You are ensuring that it has the "fuel" and the structural integrity to keep beating strong for decades to come. Don't let the "no pain, no gain" mythology rob you of your health. Real gain comes from the balance of hard work and deep, restorative peace.

**The Power of Progressive Muscle Relaxation**

Sometimes, even when we lie down to rest, our bodies remain tight. We carry the stress of the day in our shoulders, our jaws, and our chests. This residual tension keeps the heart in a "ready" state, preventing it from fully entering the recovery phase. To combat this, I want to introduce a technique called Progressive Muscle Relaxation (PMR). This is a simple but incredibly effective way to physically "shut down" the tension in your limbs and signal to your heart that the day is over. It's like flipping the breakers on an electrical panel one by one until the whole house is quiet.

Here is how you do it: Lie flat on your back in bed with your eyes closed. Start at your toes. Tense the muscles in your feet as hard as you can for five seconds, then suddenly release them. Feel the blood rush back into the area and notice the sensation of limpness. Move up to your calves and do the same—tense for five, release for ten. Continue this process through your thighs, your buttocks, your abdomen, your hands, your arms, and finally your shoulders and face. By the time you reach the top of your head, your entire body will be in a state of deep physical release. This drop in muscle tension leads to an immediate decrease in peripheral resistance, allowing your heart rate to glide down into its lowest resting state. It is a manual override for your nervous system, and it works every single time.

Practicing PMR before you fall asleep ensures that you aren't "gritting your teeth" through the night. It clears the physical slate so that your sleep can be truly restorative. Many people find that they fall asleep before they even finish the routine. That's perfectly fine! The goal is to reach that state of total let-go. When your muscles are relaxed, your heart doesn't have to work to pump blood through tight, constricted tissues. It can beat slowly and powerfully, focusing all its energy on repair rather than overcoming resistance. This is the ultimate gift you can give to your cardiovascular system.

### Reflection: Rest is Not Laziness

As we wrap up this look at recovery, I want you to sit with a very important question: Do you view rest as "laziness" or as "recovery"? In our fast-paced society, we are often made to feel guilty for taking time off. We feel like if we aren't being productive, we are falling behind. But I want you to reframe that thinking. Rest is the most productive thing you can do for your heart. Without it, your diet and your exercise are just spinning wheels. When you choose to go to bed early or take a rest day, you aren't being lazy; you are being an elite manager of your own health. You are making a high-level executive decision to prioritize the long-term viability of your most important organ.

Think about how you feel after a full eight hours of high-quality sleep. Your mind is sharper, your mood is better, and your body feels light and ready for action. That feeling is the result of a heart that has been allowed to heal. Compare that to the "foggy" feeling of a night with only five hours of sleep. That fog isn't just in your head; it's in your whole system. It's the feeling of a heart that is struggling to keep up because it never got its "quiet time." Choose the clarity. Choose the vitality. Choose the rest. Your heart has been beating for you since before you were born; the least you can do is give it a few hours of peace every night.

Take ownership you treat recovery with the respect it deserves, you'll find that your entire life improves. You'll have more energy for your family, more focus for your work, and more "heart" for everything you do. You've done the hard work of learning about diet, exercise, and anatomy. Now, do the even harder work of letting go and letting your body do what it was designed to do: heal. Your heart belongs to you, and it needs you to be its guardian during the quiet hours of the night. Sleep well, rest deeply, and I'll see you when you're recharged and ready for the next step on this journey.

# Chapter 17
## Mind Over Matter: The Psychology of Success

Imagine for a second that you are the pilot of a high-performance jet. You have the best fuel in the tank, the wings are polished to a mirror shine, and the engines are primed for a transcontinental flight. But what happens if the pilot is disoriented, fearful, or constantly second-guessing the flight path? Even the most perfect machine will eventually veer off course or, worse, suffer a mechanical failure due to the erratic demands of a panicked operator. Your body is that jet, and your mind is the pilot sitting in the cockpit. If you want to see real, lasting changes in your cardiovascular health, you have to realize that the gray matter between your ears is just as vital, but now we must address the command center. Without a focused, positive psychological foundation, even the best treadmill routine in the world will eventually feel like a chore rather than a gift.

The connection between your thoughts and your physical health is not just some "new age" concept from a California retreat; it is hard science that we are understanding better every single day here in the 1990s. When you think a thought, your brain releases a cascade of chemicals that travel throughout your entire system. If you are constantly dwelling on failure, stress, or the "inevitability" of poor health, you are essentially bathing your heart in a soup of stress hormones. Conversely, when you adopt a winner's mindset, you create a physiological environment where healing and growth can actually happen. Success in any fitness endeavor begins with a mental blueprint. You have to see the healthy version of yourself before you can inhabit that body. It is time to stop treating your mind as a passive observer of your health and start using it as the primary driver of your success.

### The Physiology of Emotion:

### When the Mind Breaks the Heart

To understand why your mindset matters so much, we need to look at a fascinating and somewhat startling condition known as Takotsubo cardiomyopathy. In common parlance, this is often called "Broken Heart Syndrome." It happens when a person experiences an overwhelming emotional event—usually something like the sudden loss of a loved one or an intense period of extreme fear. In these moments, the brain triggers a massive surge of adrenaline and other stress chemicals. This surge is so powerful that it actually causes the left ventricle of the heart to change shape. It balloons out at the bottom while staying narrow at the top, making the heart look like a traditional Japanese octopus trap (a *takotsubo*).

This physical deformity makes it incredibly difficult for the heart to pump blood effectively. People suffering from this condition often feel like they are having a massive heart attack, even though their coronary arteries might be perfectly clear. While most people recover with time and rest, this condition proves one very important point: your emotions have the power to physically reshape your organs. If a single moment of intense sadness can warp the very structure of your heart, imagine what years of low-level chronic stress and negative self-talk are doing to your cardiac grinding pressure that prevents you from reaching your full potential.

The “Broken Heart” phenomenon shows us that the heart is not just a pump; it is a sensory organ that is deeply integrated with our nervous system. Every time you tell yourself “I’ll never get in shape” or “Heart disease runs in my family, so why bother?”, you are sending a signal of defeat to your cardiac cells. This isn’t just about “feeling bad”; it’s about the chemical reality of cortisol. High levels of cortisol, the body’s primary stress hormone, lead to increased blood pressure, higher cholesterol production, and even the accumulation of dangerous visceral fat around your midsection. By changing the way you think, you are effectively changing the chemical prescription your brain writes for your heart every single morning.

### Visualization: The 90s Wellness Edge

If the mind can break the heart, it can also build it. One of the most effective tools we have in our 1990s wellness toolkit is the practice of creative visualization. High-level athletes have been using this for years. A downhill skier will close their eyes and “run” the entire course in their mind, feeling every turn and every jump before they even click into their bindings. They aren’t just daydreaming; they are “firing” the neural pathways required for success. We can apply this exact same principle to your cardiovascular health. When you visualize your heart, you shouldn’t just think of it as a generic red shape. You should picture it as a powerful, clean, and efficient engine.

Visualization works because the brain has a hard time distinguishing between a vividly imagined event and a real one.

When you sit quietly and see yourself finishing a three-mile walk with ease, your body yourself as a vibrant, energetic person who loves nutritious food, you are much more likely to make choices that align with that vision. The reason most diets and exercise plans fail isn't a lack of information; it's a lack of identity. People try to change their habits without changing the way they see themselves. They are "overweight people trying to be thin" rather than "healthy people acting like healthy people." Visualization bridges that gap.

Try this exercise: Close your eyes and imagine the blood flowing through your veins. Don't see it as a sluggish, thick fluid. See it as a bright, oxygen-rich river that is moving effortlessly through wide, flexible arteries. Imagine your heart beating with a steady, confident rhythm. Every beat is pushing life-giving nutrients to your toes, your fingertips, and your brain. Picture the walls of your heart as systemic tension. When you spend time in this mental space, you are training your autonomic nervous system to stay in a state of calm readiness rather than frantic stress.

### The Power of Positive Affirmations

Let's talk about the soundtrack playing in your head. Most of us have a "nagger" living in our minds—a voice that points out every flaw, every missed workout, and every cookie we shouldn't have eaten. This negative self-talk is a poison for your motivation. To counter it, we use positive affirmations. Now, don't roll your eyes! Affirmations aren't about lying to yourself or ignoring reality. They are about intentionally choosing the thoughts that will serve your goals. An affirmation is a short, powerful statement in the present tense that describes the person you are becoming.

"I am healthy," you say, "I am a strong person with a vibrant heart." Instead of "I hope I lose weight," you say, "I nourish my body with food that gives me energy." By repeating these phrases daily, you are literally re-wiring your brain. inspiration (moving toward what you love). Positive motivation is a much more sustainable fuel source for a long-term lifestyle change.

Consider the impact of these two different mental approaches:

- **Negative Approach:** "I have to go to the gym because I'm out of shape and my doctor is worried about my cholesterol. I hate this, but I don't want to have a heart attack."
- **Positive Affirmation Approach:** "I energy to enjoy my family."

The first person is operating out of fear. Fear is a great short-term motivator, but it's exhausting. The second person is operating out of a sense of purpose and identity. They are much more likely to stick with the program for the next twenty years because their "why" is rooted in something positive. Your heart responds to the joy of movement, not just the obligation of it. When you speak to yourself with kindness and authority, you lower the emotional barrier to entry for your daily exercise.

### Ancient Wisdom: The Stoic Heart

While the 1990s have brought us amazing breakthroughs in psychology, we can also learn a lot by looking back at the ancient world. The Stoic philosophers of Greece and Rome, like Marcus Aurelius and Epictetus, understood the "mind over matter" connection better than almost anyone. They taught that while we cannot always control what happens to us—the genes we are born with, the stress of our jobs, or the fluctuations of the economy—we have absolute control over how we react to those things. They viewed the mind as a fortress. If the fortress is strong, the chaos outside cannot harm the person within.

This Stoic approach is perfectly suited for heart health. Think about the "Type A" personality that was so often discussed in the 1980s. This is the person who is always in a hurry, always angry at traffic, and always stressed about deadlines. From a Stoic perspective, this person is allowing external events to dictate their internal state. Every time they get angry at a red light, their heart rate spikes and their blood pressure soars. They are giving away their power to a piece of colored glass on a street corner! A Stoic would say, "I cannot change the light, so why should I let it damage my heart?"

By adopting a bit of this ancient philosophy, you can protect your heart from the "micro-stressors" of daily life. When you encounter a setback—maybe you missed a week of workouts due to the flu—a Stoic doesn't descend into guilt and self-loathing. They simply acknowledge the fact, decide on the best course of action for today, and move forward. They understand that the past is unchangeable and the future is uncertain, so the only place where health can system. It keeps your "engine" from revving unnecessarily, preserving your energy for the things that actually matter.

## Common Mistakes:

### The Trap of 'Negative Motivation'

One of the biggest hurdles I see people face is the reliance on shame as a motivator. We live in a culture that often uses guilt to sell everything from gym memberships to diet sodas. You see an ad with a "perfect" body and you feel bad about yours, so you buy the product. This is shame-based motivation, and it is a recipe for failure. Shame is a "heavy" emotion. It causes your body to contract, your breathing to become shallow, and your stress levels to rise. When you exercise because you "hate" your body, you are essentially punishing yourself. How long can anyone realistically keep up a routine that feels like a punishment?

Another common mistake is the "all or nothing" mentality. This is the psychological trap where one small mistake leads to a total collapse of the plan. You eat one piece of birthday cake, and your brain says, "Well, the whole day is ruined! I might as well eat the pizza and skip the walk." This happens because we tie our self-worth to our perfection. We need to reframe our thinking: health is a practice, not a destination. You are not "on" or "off" a plan. You are simply a person making a series of choices. One choice doesn't define the rest of your life. If you make a choice that doesn't align with your goals, the very next choice is an opportunity to get back on track. This cognitive reframing removes the massive emotional weight that often accompanies diet and exercise.

Finally, many people ignore the emotional roots of their habits. We often use food or sedentary behavior as a way to "numb out" from stress or emotional pain. If you don't address the reason why you are reaching for that high-fat snack in the middle of the night, no amount of willpower will save you in the long run. You have to be willing to look at the "why" behind your "what." Are you eating because you're hungry, or because you're lonely? Are you skipping your walk because you're tired, or because you're afraid of failing? Identifying these emotional triggers allows you to find better ways to cope that don't involve damaging your heart. Motivation is a muscle, and like any muscle, it needs the right nutrients—in this case, honesty and self-compassion.

### Action Step 1: Your Daily Health Affirmation

It is time to put these concepts into action. The first step in your mental makeover is to create a personal health affirmation. I want you to get a piece of paper or a small index card. Write down a single sentence that reflects the healthy person you are becoming. Remember the rules: present tense, positive, and personal. Do not use words like "won't," "can't," or "don't." Focus entirely on what you **are** and what you **can** do.

Here are a few examples to get your brain moving:

1. "I am a person who values my heart and fuels my body with vitality."
2. "Every day, my heart grows stronger and my energy increases."
3. "I love the feeling of my lungs breathing deeply and my blood flowing freely."
4. "I am disciplined, capable, and worthy of a long, healthy life."

Once you have written your affirmation, place it somewhere you will see it every single morning. Maybe it goes on the bathroom mirror, or maybe you tape it to the dashboard of your car. Read it out loud. Yes, out loud! There is something powerful about hearing your own voice speak your truth. Say it with conviction. Even if you don't fully believe it yet, keep saying it. You are planting a seed in your subconscious mind. With daily repetition, that seed will grow into a belief, and that belief will eventually become your reality. You are the author of your own story; make sure you are writing a hero's journey, not a tragedy.

### Action Step 2: The Two-Minute Heart Visualization

The second part of your action plan is to dedicate just two minutes a day to a specific heart visualization. This is best done in the morning before you get out of bed or in the evening right before you fall asleep. Sit or lie comfortably and close your eyes. Take three deep, slow breaths, feeling your belly rise and fall. This signals to your nervous system that it is time to relax.

Now, bring your internal "camera" inside your chest. See your heart as a magnificent, muscular organ. It is a deep, healthy red, and it is glowing with a soft, warm light. Watch it contract and expand with effortless power. See the valves opening and closing with perfect precision, like the doors of a world-class hotel. Visualize the blood as a sparkling, clear stream of energy that is carrying away any waste and bringing in everything your cells need to thrive. If you have been worried about a specific issue, like high blood pressure, imagine the walls of your arteries becoming smooth and flexible, like high-quality silk. See the pressure dropping to a perfect, calm level.

Don't rush this. Really try to *feel* the strength of your heart. Imagine that with every beat, a wave of calm and health is spreading from your chest out to the rest of your body. You are not just a collection of parts; you are a unified system, and your heart is the conductor of the orchestra. After two minutes, take one more deep breath, open your eyes, and carry that feeling of "internal strength" with you into your day. This simple practice reduces the ambient stress on your heart and reinforces your commitment to your health goals.

### Action Step 3: Journaling Your 'Why'

The third and perhaps most important step is to spend some time journaling about your "Why." Motivation is a fickle friend; it shows up when you're excited and disappears when you're tired or busy. To stay consistent, you need a deep, emotional reason for why you want to be healthy. This reason has to be bigger than "I want to look good in a swimsuit" or "I want to lower my numbers." Those are fine goals, but they rarely have the "teeth" to keep you going through the hard times.

Ask yourself: What will a healthy heart allow youed. Maybe it's the confidence to take that hiking trip you've always dreamed of. Maybe it's the peace of mind that comes from knowing you aren't a burden to your family. Whatever it is, write it down in vivid detail. Describe the sights, the sounds, and especially the feelings of that future success. When you have a clear, emotional "Why," the "How" becomes much easier. On the days when you don't feel like exercising, you can look back at your journal and remind yourself what you are actually working for. You aren't just "walking"; you are "walking so I can see my daughter walk down the aisle." That is the kind of motivation that lasts a lifetime.

In addition to your "Why," use your journal to identify one "negative self-talk" habit. We all have one. Maybe yours is "I'm just naturally lazy" or "I've always been the 'big' one in the family." Write that sentence down, then draw a big "X" through it. Below it, write the replacement thought. If the old thought was "I'm too old to change," the new thought is "I am gaining wisdom and strength every day." Whenever you catch that old, negative voice starting up, mentally say "STOP" and replace it with your new, positive statement. You are the gatekeeper of your mind. Don't let any "unauthorized personnel" in to mess with your success.

### The Chemical Reward of Success

As you begin to master these psychological tools, something amazing will happen. You will start to feel a shift in your physical energy. This isn't just "power of suggestion"; it is the result of your body's chemistry changing. When you move from a state of chronic stress and "negative motivation" into a state of positive focus and visualization, your brain starts producing more dopamine and endorphins. These are the body's "feel-good" chemicals. They act as natural painkillers and mood elevators. They also happen to be great for your heart, as they help to relax the blood vessels and improve circulation.

This creates a "virtuous cycle." Because you feel better mentally, you have more energy to exercise and eat well. Because you are exercising and eating well, your body feels better. Because your body feels better, your mind stays positive. This is the exact opposite of the "downward spiral" that so many people find themselves in. The hardest part is simply getting the wheel to turn the other way for the first time. By using affirmations and visualization, you are giving that wheel its first big push. You aren't waiting for your body to change before you feel good; you are feeling good so that your body **can** change.

Remember, your thoughts create your reality. This isn't a metaphor heart that is strong, resilient, and long-lasting, you must provide it with a mental environment that supports those qualities. You have the power to choose your thoughts. Choose the ones that lead to life.

### Reflection: Do You Believe You Deserve to Be Healthy?

Before we move forward into the next phase of our journey, I want you to take a moment for some honest self-reflection. Sit quietly and ask yourself this question: **"Do I truly believe I deserve to be healthy and vibrant?"** It sounds like a simple question, but for many of us, the answer is buried under layers of old stories, past failures, and feelings of unworthiness. Some of us have been told for so long that we are "unathletic" or "genetically cursed" that we have started to believe it. We might even be subconsciously sabotaging our own efforts because we don't feel like we "belong" in the world of healthy, fit people.

Let me tell you right now: you deserve a healthy heart. You deserve to wake up with energy. You deserve to feel strong in your own skin. This is your birthright as a human being. Your heart has been working tirelessly for you since before you were born, never asking for a break, never complaining. It believes in you! It is ready to get stronger the moment you give it the chance. Don't let old, dusty ideas about yourself stand in the way of your future. If you failed in the past, that was just data. It wasn't a judgment on your character. Today is a new day, and you are a new person with new tools and a new mindset.

You have the affirmations, the visualization, and the "Why." You have the ancient wisdom of the Stoics and the modern science of the 90s. Most importantly, you have the pilot's seat. Your mind is ready to lead, and your heart is ready to follow. Let's make this flight a long and beautiful one. You have everything you need to succeed. Now, go out there and live like the healthy person you already are in your mind. The rest of your body will catch up soon enough.

These three changes—the daily affirmation, the two-minute visualization, and the "Why" journaling—applied consistently, will transform your relationship with your health. Your heart belongs to you, and today, you have finally taken full command of the ship. Stay focused, stay positive, and keep moving forward. I'll see you in the next chapter as we turn these mental victories into a lifelong plan for success.

# Chapter 18
## *Goal Setting for a Lifetime of Health*

Say, you want to live longer? How about taking steps to improve your body through diet and exercise and an understanding of your heart as well as the human heart altogether throughout the ages? Well you've come to the right place, let me tell you. We have spent plenty of time discussing the nitty-gritty of cholesterol, the burn of the aerobic zone, and the mental grit required to stay the course. But here is a cold, hard truth: a dream without a plan is just a wish. You can visualize a healthy heart until the cows come home, but if you don't have a roadmap to get there, you're just spinning your wheels in the driveway. We need to turn those high-energy intentions into a concrete strategy that lasts not just for a week or a month, but for the rest of your life.

Think of your heart as a high-performance engine in a classic muscle car. You wouldn't just drive it into the ground and hope for the best, would you? No, you'd have deserves that same level of tactical precision. In this chapter, we are going to bridge the gap between "wanting" to be healthy and "being" healthy by using a system that works. We're moving away from vague promises and moving toward a structural framework that makes success almost inevitable. It's about taking that big, intimidating mountain of "fitness" and carving out a nice, paved path right to the top.

## The Training Effect: Reshaping the Pump

Before we get into the "how-to" of goal setting, I want to talk about why consistency is your best friend from a purely biological standpoint. In the medical world, we talk about something called the **Training Effect**. This isn't just a fancy way of saying you're getting in shape; it refers to the actual, physical adaptations your heart makes when you challenge it regularly over a long period. When you commit to a long-term plan, you aren't just losing a few pounds. You are literally remodeling your internal architecture.

When you perform aerobic exercise consistently, your heart undergoes **cardiac hypertrophy**. Now, don't let that big word scare you. While some types of heart enlargement are bad, the kind that comes from exercise is a sign of a true athlete. The walls of your left ventricle—the chamber responsible for pumping oxygen-rich blood to the rest of your body—become thicker and stronger. More importantly, the chamber itself can actually hold more blood. What does this mean for your daily life? It means your heart becomes more efficient. Because it can move more blood with one pump, it doesn't have to beat as often when you're sitting on the couch or sleeping. This is why highly effect doesn't happen overnight. It is the result of thousands of small, repeated signals sent to your heart telling it that it needs to be better. If you exercise once and then quit for two weeks, your heart has no reason to change. It only adapts when it realizes that this "challenge" is the new normal. That is why a structured plan is the only way to trigger these deep, structural changes that add years to your life.

### The SMART Strategy for Cardiac Success

In the business world of the 90s, everyone is talking about **SMART** goals. It's a framework that has helped CEOs turn companies around, and it's going to do the same for your heart. The reason most people fail at their health goals is that they are too vague. They say, "I want to get healthy" or "I need to exercise more." Those aren't goals; they're pipe dreams. To get real results, your goals need to be sharp and defined. Let's break down the SMART acronym so you can apply it to your own life starting today.

- **Specific:** Your goal should be clear and unambiguous. Instead of "I want to walk more," say "I will walk for 30 minutes at a brisk pace." You need to know exactly what the finish line looks like.

- **Measurable:** If you can't track it, you can't progress at the end of the week and say, "Yes, I did exactly what I set out to do."

- **Achievable:** This is where many people trip up. They haven't exercised in ten years, but they decide they're going to run a marathon next month. That's a recipe for injury and discouragement. Pick a goal that challenges you but is within the realm of possibility for your current fitness level.

- **Relevant:** Make sure your goal actually matters to *your* heart. If your blood pressure is high, a goal related to reducing salt or increasing aerobic activity is highly relevant. Your goal should align with the specific health outcomes you want to see.

- **Time-bound:** Every goal needs a deadline. “Someday” is not a day of the week. Give yourself a thirty-day window to achieve a specific milestone. This creates a sense of healthy urgency and keeps you from procrastinating.

By using this framework, you take the guesswork out of your routine. You wake up in the morning knowing exactly what you plan is set in stone, you don’t have to rely on fleeting bursts of motivation. You just follow the map.

### The Power of Mini-Victories

Once you have your big SMART goal, the secret to staying on track is the **Mini-Victory System**. Let’s say your goal is to lose ten pounds and lower your resting heart rate by five beats per minute over the next three months. That’s a great goal, but it’s a long way off. If you only celebrate when you reach the final destination, you’re going to get bored and frustrated along the way. You need to break that big goal into tiny, bite-sized pieces that you can win every single week.

A mini-victory is a small, manageable win that keeps your momentum moving salad instead of fries three times.” These might seem insignificant, but they are the bricks that build the fortress of your health. Every time you achieve a mini-victory, your brain gets a little hit of dopamine. This reinforces the behavior and makes you want to do it again. You are essentially training yourself to enjoy the process of being healthy. Success breeds success. When you stack enough of these small wins on top of each other, the big goal starts to take care of itself.

Think of it like a staircase. You don't jump from the bottom floor to the second story in one leap. You take one step at a time. If you focus only on the top of the stairs, you might trip. But if you focus on just landing your foot firmly on the next step, you'll be at the top before you know it. The Mini-Victory System turns the "grind" of lifestyle change into a series of rewarding milestones. It keeps your spirits high and your heart pumping with confidence.

### The History of the Resolution: Why We Fail

Humans have been making promises to improve often credited with being the first people to make New Year's resolutions. At the start of each year, they would make promises to their gods to pay their debts and return borrowed farm equipment. If they kept their word, their gods would look upon them with favor for the coming year. If they failed, well, let's just say they didn't want to find out.

Later, the Romans continued this tradition by making sacrifices to the god Janus, the two-faced deity who looked both backward into the past year and forward into the future. But here is the interesting part: throughout history, these resolutions were usually about external actions—paying back money or performing rituals. It wasn't until much later that resolutions became about internal "self-improvement" like diet and exercise. And that is where we started to run into trouble.

The reason modern New Year's resolutions fail so spectacularly—usually by the second week of February—is that they are based on *guilt* rather than *strategy*. People wait until they feel terrible about their holiday overindulgence, and then they make a massive, sweeping change that they can't possibly sustain. They try to change everything at once without any understanding of how habits are actually formed. They treat their health like a temporary project rather than a lifelong commitment. By looking at the history of these failures, we can learn a vital lesson: lasting change doesn't come from a once-a-year burst of enthusiasm. It comes from a daily, deliberate system of goal setting and tracking.

### Common Pitfalls in Goal Setting

Even with the best intentions, it's easy to fall into a few common traps that can derail your progress. One of the biggest mistakes is setting **vague goals**. If you tell yourself you want to "eat better," what does that actually mean? Does it mean less fat? More fiber? Fewer calories? Without a specific target, your brain doesn't know how to execute foods you've always bought. Be specific!

Another trap is the **"Too Much, Too Soon"** syndrome. I see this all the time at the local gym in January. People who haven't moved faster than a brisk walk in years suddenly decide they are going to do an hour of high-impact aerobics every single day. By the end of the first week, their knees are screaming, their back is out of whack, and they are so exhausted they can barely function at work. They quit because the "cost" of the goal is too high. Remember, your heart is a muscle that needs to be coaxed into strength, not beaten into it.

# Chapter 19

## *The Future of Your Heart: A Lifelong Commitment*

So, we have reached the finish line. Or have we? If you have been following along, you probably realize by now that in the world of cardiovascular fitness, there is no such thing as a final destination. You do not just "arrive" at a healthy heart and then park the car for good. If you stop up your sneakers and get into that target zone. But the real test begins tomorrow morning when you wake up and decide to>

Think about the commitment you have made. Many people treat health like a summer blockbuster. They show up for the opening weekend, get all excited by the special effects, and then they forget about it by the time the next season rolls around. That is not how we do things here. We are looking for a lifelong partnership between your mind and your body. This the "get fit quick" schemes that clutter the television airwaves. Instead, you have embraced a philosophy of steady, sustainable growth. It is about being better this year than you were last year, and staying that way until you are eighty, ninety, or beyond talk about a concept called **Cardiac Reserve**. This is one of those medical terms that sounds complicated but is actually quite intuitive. Imagine your heart is a bank account. Every time you go for a brisk walk, choose a baked potato over french fries, or manage your stress with deep breathing, you are making a deposit. Your cardiac reserve is the difference between the rate at which your heart pumps blood when you are resting and its maximum capacity for pumping blood during intense physical exertion. It to shrink that margin. If you do not exercise, your heart becomes less efficient. It has to beat faster just to do basic tasks like climbing a flight of stairs or carrying groceries. When a real stressor comes along—maybe a bout of the flu, a sudden emotional shock, or a period of intense physical labor—a person with low cardiac reserve might find themselves in serious trouble. Their heart simply does not have the extra "oomph" to meet the demand.

By staying active and keeping your weight in check, you are expanding that reserve. You are building a buffer. A fit individual might have a cardiac reserve that is four or five times their resting output. This means that if life throws a curveball, their car. You might usually drive at fifty-five miles per hour, but it is nice to know that if you need to pass someone on the highway, you have the horsepower to do it safely. Building this reserve is the best insurance policy you can ever buy for yourself. It protects you against the inevitable wear and tear of time.

This reserve is not just about surviving emergencies, though. It is about the quality of your daily existence. When you have a high cardiac the garden without feeling like you need a week to recover. You are literally more alive because your heart is capable of delivering more oxygen and nutrients to every cell in your body with less effort. That is the ultimate goal of this entire program: to make you more capable of enjoying the world around you.

### The Annual Heart Review

Now, how do we make sure we are actually maintaining this reserve? We need a system. In the business world, people have annual performance reviews to see if they are meeting their goals. Why should your health be any different? I recommend that every person reading this book implements what I call the **Annual Heart Review**. This is a specific time, perhaps on your birthday or every New Year's Day, where you sit down and take a hard look at the data. You cannot manage what you do not measure, and you certainly cannot improve what you ignore. During your Annual Heart Review, you should look at three main areas: your physical metrics, your habits, and your goals for the coming year. This is not about beating yourself up if you had a few bad weeks during the holidays. It is about looking at the big picture. Are you stronger than you were twelve months ago? Is your resting pulse staying in a healthy range? Let's break down how to conduct this review properly.

1. **Analyze the Numbers:** Look back at your logs. If you have been tracking your exercise, look at the frequency and intensity. Did you hit your target heart rate consistently? Check your weight and, if possible, your blood pressure and cholesterol levels from your last doctor's visit. Trends matter more than single data points. If your blood pressure has been creeping up over the last three years, that is a signal that you need to adjust your sodium intake or increase your aerobic activity.
2. **Evaluate the Kitchen:** Be honest about your diet. Have old habits started to sneak back in? Maybe you started out the year eating oatmeal every morning but lately you have been grabbing a donut on the way to work. It happens to the best of us. Use the review to recalibrate. Go back to the basics of high-fiber, low-saturated-fat eating. Remind yourself why you made those changes in the first place.
3. **Assess Your Energy:** How do you feel? This is a subjective measure, but it is incredibly important. Do you have the stamina to get through your day? Are you sleeping well? Often, a decline in "feeling good" is the first sign that our cardiovascular health is slipping. If you feel sluggish, it might be time to shake up your exercise routine.
4. **Update Your Equipment:** Check your shoes. If you have been walking or running regularly, your

sneakers are probably worn out after a year. Old shoes can lead to joint pain, which gives you an excuse to stop exercising. Spend the money on a good pair of athletic shoes. It is a small investment that pays huge dividends in consistency.

The beauty of the Annual Heart Review is that it prevents you from drifting. Most people do not wake up one day and decide to be unhealthy. They just stop paying attention. They skip a workout here, eat a greasy meal there, and before they know it, five years have passed and they have gained twenty pounds and lost their breath walking to the mailbox. By checking in once a year, you catch those small slips before they become permanent landslides. You stay in the driver's seat of your own life.

### A Vision of the Future

As we sit here in the early 1990s, the world is changing fast. We are seeing incredible leaps in medical technology and our understanding of the human body. It is exciting to think about what the next century will bring for heart health. We are already seeing the beginnings of more sophisticated ways to monitor our internal workings. While we currently rely on manual pulse checks and blood pressure cuffs at the pharmacy, imagine a future where we might have even more precise tools right in our own homes.

The 21st century will likely bring new discoveries in genetics and nutrition that will make our current advice look like the stone age. However, no matter how much technology advances, the fundamentals will never change. The human heart is a muscle. It needs to be worked. The human body is a biological machine. It needs clean fuel. Even if they invent a pill that mimics the effects of exercise, it will never replace the mental clarity and the sense of accomplishment that comes.

We are also seeing a shift in how we think about the mind-body connection. In the past, doctors mostly looked at the heart as a mechanical pump. If it broke, you tried to fix the parts. But we are learning more every day about how stress, loneliness, and even our sense of purpose affects our cardiovascular system. The heart truly is the center of our emotional lives as much as our physical ones. Looking forward, the most successful health strategies will be the ones that treat the whole person, not just the organ. By taking care of your stress and building strong relationships, you are doing just as much for your arteries as you are by eating your vegetables.

I believe we are entering an era of the "empowered patient." You are no longer someone who just waits for a doctor to tell you what is wrong. You are the primary caretaker of your own health. You have the information. You have the tools. You have the motivation. The future not have to be a victim of your genetics or your environment. You can choose a different path.

## Your Lifelong Action Plan

I want to leave you with some very specific steps to take as you close this book and move into the rest of your life. This is not a "goodbye," but a "see you on the trail." We have built a foundation together, and now it is time for you to build the house. These three actions will help solidify everything you have learned and ensure that your commitment to your heart remains ironclad.

### Step 1: Review Your Initial Heart Log

Go back to the very first chapter of this book. Find that log where you recorded your starting weight, your resting heart rate, and how you felt after a ten-minute walk. Compare those numbers to where you are today. It is easy to forget how far you have come when you are focused on how much further you want to go. Seeing the physical proof of your progress is the best way to stay motivated. If your resting pulse has dropped from eighty beats per minute to seventy, that is a massive victory! That means your heart is beating 14,400 fewer times every single day. Think about the wear and tear you are saving. Celebrate that progress. You earned it.

### Step 2: Write a Letter to Your Future Self

This might sound a little bit cheesy, but stay with me. I want you to sit down and write a letter to yourself that you will open exactly one year from today. In this letter, tell your future self why you started this journey. Remind yourself of how much better you feel now that you have more energy and less stress. Describe the goals you have met and the ones you are still working on. Tell your future self that you are worth the effort. Seal it in an envelope, write the date on the front, and put it somewhere safe—maybe with your holiday decorations or in your filing cabinet. When you open it next year, it will serve as a powerful reminder of the promises you made to yourself.

### Step 3: Share the Wealth

The best way to keep what, or a friend—and share one specific thing you have learned from this book. Maybe you can explain the importance of fiber, or show them how to take their own pulse. Better yet, invite them to go for a walk with you. When you teach someone else, you reinforce the knowledge in your own mind. Plus, health is contagious. When people see you looking better and having more energy, they will want to know your secret. By being a role model, you are not just helping yourself; you are potentially saving the lives of the people you care about most. There is no greater legacy than that.

## The Marathon Mentality

As you move forward, remember that heart health is a marathon, not a sprint. There will be days when you don't feel like exercising. There will be parties where the buffet is full of fried foods and high-fat desserts. There will be weeks when stress at work makes you want to crawl into a hole and eat a bag of potato chips. That is okay. You are human. The key is not to be perfect; the key is to be consistent over the long haul.

If you fall off the wagon, don't spend three days beating yourself up about it. Just get back on. The very next meal is an opportunity to make a better choice. The very next morning is an opportunity to go for a walk. A single "bad" day cannot undo months of hard work unless you let it turn into a "bad" month or a "bad" year. Keep your eyes on the horizon. Think about where you want to be ten, twenty, and thirty years from now. You want to be the person who is still active, still sharp, and still enjoying every beat of their heart.

But your heart is the only thing you truly own from the moment you are born until the moment you die. It has been working for you every second of every day, usually without you even noticing. It is a faithful servant. Isn't it time you treated it with the respect it deserves? You have the knowledge now. You know how to eat, how to move, and how to think in a way that supports this incredible organ. The rest is up to you.

## Common Mistakes to Avoid

Before we wrap things up, I want to warn you about a few traps that people often fall into once they finish a program like this. Knowing about these ahead of time will help you stay on track when things get tough.

- **The "I'm Done" Trap:** This is the biggest mistake of all. People hit their target weight or lower their cholesterol to a healthy level and think they have "finished" their health journey. They go back to their old ways, and within a few months, all their progress is gone. Remember, you are never "done." Health is a daily practice, just like brushing your teeth or taking out the trash.
- **The "All or Nothing" Mentality:** Some people think that if they can't do a full forty-five-minute workout, there is no point in doing anything at all. This is completely false. If you only have ten minutes, take a ten-minute walk. It still counts! Doing something is always infinitely better than doing nothing. Don't let perfection be the enemy of progress.
- **The Information Silo:** Some people learn all this great information and then keep it to themselves. They don't talk about their goals or their struggles with anyone else. This makes it much harder to stay accountable. Share your journey. Find a workout buddy. Join a walking club. Having a community makes the lifestyle much easier to maintain.
- **Ignoring the Subtle Signs:** Sometimes our bodies try to tell us things in very quiet ways. Maybe your joints are a little stiffer, or you're feeling a bit more winded than usual. Don't ignore these small changes. They are your heart's way of asking for a little more attention. Pay attention to the whispers so you don't have to deal with the screams.

### Reflecting on Your Journey

Take a second to think back to when you first picked up this book. How has your view of your heart changed? In the beginning, you might have seen it as just a pump, or perhaps you didn't think about it at all. Now, I hope you see it as a dynamic, living part of you that responds to every choice you make. I hope you feel a sense of awe at its complexity and its resilience. It is truly a miracle of biological engineering.

What are you going to do to ensure that this isn't just a "phase"? We have all had phases—the phase where we tried to learn a new language, the phase where we took up pottery, the phase where we decided to wear neon colors. Health cannot be a phase. It has to be your new normal. Think about the habits you have you hate running but love swimming, then swim! If you hate broccoli but love spinach, then eat spinach! The best heart-healthy lifestyle is the one that you actually like living.

You have learned about the history of the heart, from the ancient Egyptians who thought it was the seat of the soul to the modern scientists who map every artery. You have learned about the role of cholesterol and the power of fiber. You have learned how to calculate your target heart rate and how to cool down properly after a workout. This is a complete toolkit. You are now your own best health advocate. You don't need to wait for a doctor's permission to live a better life. You have the power to make that choice every single day.

As we close this chapter and this book, I want you to take a deep breath. Feel your lungs expand. Feel your heart beat in your chest. That rhythm is the sound of life. It is the most beautiful sound in the world. It is the sound of your past, your present, and your future. Take care of that rhythm. Protect it. Cherish it. Because your heart belongs to you, and it is the only one you will ever have.

I am proud of the work you have done. I am excited for the life you are going to lead. Go out there and make every heartbeat count. Whether you are walking through your neighborhood, cooking a healthy meal for your family, or just sitting quietly and appreciating the gift of health, know that you are doing the right thing. You are living proof that it is never too late to start, and it is always the right time to keep going. Here is to your heart, your health, and your long, vibrant life. You've got this!

## Final Thoughts for the Road

The 90s are a decade of energy and optimism. We are looking toward a new millennium with high hopes and big dreams. But those dreams are only possible if we have the physical vitality to pursue them. By focusing on your heart health, you are setting the stage for everything else you want to achieve. A strong heart gives you the courage to take risks, the stamina to work hard, and the longevity to see your dreams come to fruition.

Don't let the noise of the world distract you from what is important. There will always be a new gadget to buy, a new show to watch, or a new reason to stay on the couch. But none of those things can provide the deep, lasting satisfaction of knowing that you are taking care of your body. When you feel that surge of energy during a morning walk, or that sense of lightness after a healthy meal, remember that feeling. That is the feeling of success. That is the feeling of a heart that is being loved and respected.

Stay curious. Keep learning. The world of health and fitness is always evolving, and you should evolve with it. Read articles, talk to experts, and stay open to new ideas. But always come back to the fundamentals we have discussed here. If it sounds too good to be true, it probably is. If it promises results without effort, it is a lie. The real secret to a healthy heart is no secret at all: it is the daily commitment to moving your body and fueling it with care.

You are part of a growing movement of people who are taking charge of their lives. You are not alone on this path. There are millions of others who are making the same choices, facing the same struggles, and celebrating the same victories. Look for them. Support them. And let them support you. Together, we can change the health of our entire society, one heart at a time.

So, one last time: get out there and move! Your heart is waiting for its next workout. Your body is waiting for its next healthy meal. And your future is waiting for you to show up and claim it. It has been a pleasure to go on this journey with you. Now, the real adventure begins. Keep that pulse strong, keep that spirit high, and remember that every single day is a gift. Make the most of it. Your heart will thank you for it, today, tomorrow, and for all the years to come. You are ready. You are capable. And most importantly, you are worth it. Good luck, and happy trails!

# Appendix/Reference Materials


1. Women Coming of Age with Jane Fonda's Prime Time Workout, Jane Fonda, Mignon McCarthy, S&S Publishing, 1984
2. Getting Strong: A Women's Guide to Realizing Her Physical Potential, Kathryn Lance, Bantam Books, 1979
3. Fully Fit in 60 Minutes a Week: The Complete Shape-up Programme for Women, Susanne O'Sullivan, Thorson's Publishing, 1984
4. Weider Book of Bodybuilding for Women, Joe and Betty Weider, Contemporary Books, 1981
5. Plyometrics: Explosive Power Training, James C. Radcliffe, Robert C. Farentinos, Human Kinetics Publishing, 1985
6. The Woman Doctor's Diet for Women: Balanced Deficit Dieting and the Brand New Re-start Diet, Barbara Edelstein, Prentice-Hall, 1977
7. 35 Plus Diet for Women, Jean Perry Spodnik, Barbara Gibbons, Souvenir Press Ltd., 1988
8. Dr. Morrison's Heart-Saver Program: A Natural, Scientifically Tested Plan for the Prevention of Arteriosclerosis, Heart Attack, and Stroke, Lester M. Morrison, Nancy Nugent, St. Martin's Press, 1983
9. The American Heart Association: Heartbook, American Heart Association, Dutton Adult, 1980
10. The Living Heart Diet, Michael Debakey, Simon & Shuster, 1986
11. Fighting Heart Disease: The History of The British Heart Foundation 1961-1988, David N. Matthews, The British Heart Foundation, 1990
12. The Heart Test: The Arizona Heart Institute Program for the Detection, Prevention, and Treatment of Heart Disease, Edward B. Diethrich, Simon & Shuster, 1981
13. And revised in 2025/2026 with internet research

# About the Author

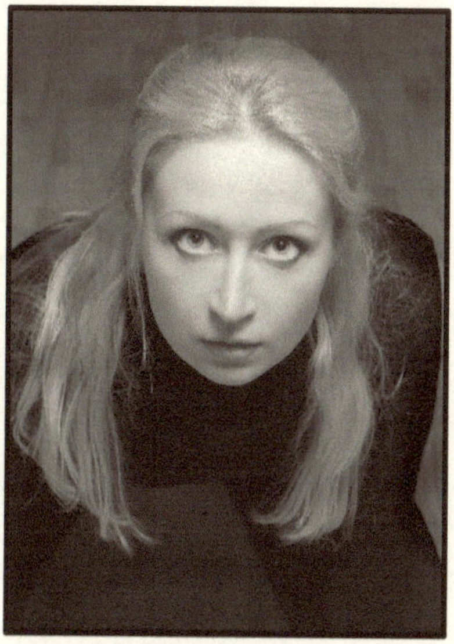

A Southern California girl from the Garden Grove suburbs who began her obsession with creative writing as a student in her elementary school circa 1970s, Marsena Shane began her literary career as soon as she graduated high school and gained her first job, a local book store clerk, before a women's fitness tutor introduced her to a New York publisher at Critic's Choice Paperbacks who published her first novella in mass market paperback, *Sweet Dreams, Lady Moon*. She became both a ghost writer and a work-for-hire, publishing her own series of fitness self-help books soon after, starting with *Great Legs in Six Weeks* (1988) which became *The Easy Way to Great Legs,* as well as *Nancy: A Reagan Biography* and subsequent works of fiction such as *June Park* and *The Martian Coal Miner*. Currently, Ms. Shane lives in Northern California with her many beloved cats, and continues to obsess with physical fitness.

www.ingramcontent.com/pod-product-compliance
Lightning Source LLC
LaVergne TN
LVHW090357210926
848480LV00002B/366